DEDICATION

⁓

THIS BOOK IS FOR JILL,
CAROLINE'S GODMOTHER

AND FOR CAROLINE'S "CARD GIRLS":
ANNA, FRANCES, HELEN, KATE, KERRIE,
SALLY AND SARAH

How far is it to London Bridge?
My Caroline would ask
As day by day we journeyed on
A long and weary task.
We laughed sometimes along the way
At other times we cried.
Fear dogged our footsteps every day
of AIDS and life denied.
When London Bridge hove into sight,
then Caroline and I
knew she could lay her burden down,
Her time had come to die.
At London Bridge she rests in peace
Soothed gently by the waves,
From AIDS cruel clutches now released
My daughter young and brave.
The rushing tide for no-one waits,
It swirls and hurries past
Bearing Tarry's spirit to the gates
Of new life, free at last.
I cannot reach my Caroline
Although I feel her near
In rock pools clear as crystal wine
I see her face so dear.
Sleep well, my daring, darling one,
Your beauty all restored
And come for me when my life's done
On London Bridge's shore.

Joan Hurley

Contents

ᴣ

Acknowledgments

My most sincere and special thanks are due to:

Doctor Philip Kennedy O.P. for his encouragement and sound advice on the early drafts of this book.

Janine Nelson for her meticulous typing and presentation of the manuscript.

Jane Waterton for her regular encouraging phone calls and letters of comfort to me throughout the time of writing.

My editor, Marg Bowman, for her thoughtful and sensitive changes and suggestions.

. . . And most of all to my husband Frank for his wisdom and patience and for understanding my need to write this book, and to my children for agreeing to it all.

PREFACE

When Caroline first came to see me she had just been discharged from hospital after treatment for an AIDS-related illness.

An exuberant and adventurous young woman and a committed traveler to the world's out-of-the-way places, she had come to talk to me about loss. In the next few years we were to talk of many things. I came to know her well: to appreciate her brightness of spirit, her wry sense of humor and her defiant courage.

The first diagnosis of AIDS in a woman was recorded in 1982. Just 10 years later, the World Health Organisation estimated that 15,000 women per week were infected worldwide. As a conservative estimate, WHO also suggests that by the year 2000, forty million people worldwide will be infected. At least half of these will be women.

Figures such as these are numbing to the mind. They do not bring home to us the reality of this devastating illness nor its consequences for those affected by the virus. What we need are personal stories. *How Far is it to London Bridge*, written by Caroline's mother, shares with us the personal story of living this experience. It is not just about loss, but also about love and support and understanding.

It can be very difficult to handle the strong emotions that are the usual response to a life-threatening illness. Caroline, like others in her situation, could at times be assailed by feelings of grief, anger, anxiety or depression.

One of the harshest aspects of HIV/AIDS is that it is primarily an illness of young adulthood. It strikes at a time of life which is generally the most vigorous and productive: a time of life when there is still much to plan for, to hope for and to achieve. For Caroline it was a great personal loss that she could no longer continue the travels she had begun at 19. She had an immense curiosity about the world and its inhabitants. Her gift for friendship enabled her to experience the family life of nomadic hill people in Tibet and the culture of villagers in South America.

As a woman with HIV, Caroline also had to confront the difficulties surrounding the issue of having children. It is possible, but by no means the rule, for HIV infection to be transmitted from mother to child. As yet we have neither vaccine to protect against infection nor cure for the disease itself. Caroline's personal choice was to have no children .

Responses to life-threatening illness have much in common, but there are additional burdens when the illness is HIV/AIDS. This is due in part to the complications of the disease itself and the treatments. But in part it is to do with community attitudes to people living with HIV/AIDS.

Although attitudes are slowly changing, there is nevertheless a stigma attached to HIV infection. HIV/AIDS is a life-threatening viral infection. We forget this fact when we add to it connotations of guilt and innocence. When we divide people living with AIDS into categories based on how they became infected and then behave differently towards them, we charge the illness with a dimension of uninformed and damaging prejudice.

Caroline had her own battles with the prejudiced. These she won with the flair of defiant courage. In all of this she was sustained and encouraged by what she herself called "the security of family and friends." All of us need loving and caring relationships with others to sustain us. In particular, when having to cope with the enormous stresses of terminal illness, being supported by those we love and trust can add immeasurably to quality of life.

Sadly and unjustly, however, fear and prejudice can diminish the quality of life for many of the people throughout the world who are living with AIDS.

For Caroline, as the disease progressed, there were periods of significant emotional and behavioral change: times when her confusional state was such that she hardly knew what she was doing. Though this was by no means usual for her, such episodes were bewildering and sad for Caroline as they were too for the family and friends who cared for and loved her. HIV infection can affect the central nervous system, causing altered psychological states and behaviors. Some opportunistic infections to which people with HIV are susceptible also cause changes in brain function and behavior, as can the powerful drugs needed to treat such infections.

We need to look with clear eyes at the impact that HIV/AIDS has now on all our lives. We need to be informed. We also need individual stories: we need them to remind us as people how much more alike we are than different – of how little separates one from another, in our human condition.

How Far is it to London Bridge is one of these individual stories. It is a candid human sharing of the impact of AIDS on Caroline and the family and friends who were deeply committed to caring for her. It reminds us of the important need for the best of our human attributes: love, understanding and compassionate care in the face of illness and death.

Donna Collidge
Psychologist, Melbourne

Chapter 1

ఌ

The Journey Begins

It was a beautiful, sunny, spring morning full of the promise of another lovely Melbourne day – but not for us. What I was about to hear would shatter the beauty of that morning irrevocably.

I had not slept very much at all that night, as I was extremely worried about Caroline's state of health. I had been worried for some months, but particularly so at that point, because she seemed to be very ill indeed and nothing was being done about it, or that's how it appeared to me. My husband, Frank, who was lying beside me, and must have been aware of my agitated tossing and turning, took my hand and asked me if I was awake. Of course I was.

"It's about Caroline, isn't it?" I asked.

It was seven o'clock on the morning of Thursday, October 13, 1988.

"Darling," he said, "I have something to tell you. But before I do, you must promise not to panic, you must not react, you must not say anything to anyone at all. You see, Caroline has AIDS. She is to be admitted to Fairfield Hospital this morning."

AIDS, AIDS, AIDS screamed through every inch of my being. This was the first I knew about Caroline having AIDS, and not just HIV, but full-blown AIDS. The sun went out, the sky went black, and I curled up into a ball and wailed in that suppressed almost silent way of a nightmare. Then I suddenly sprang out of bed, flew to the bathroom and vomited, after which I raced to the phone beside the bed and immediately rang my sister and told her. In short, I did all the things that I was specifically asked not to do. I couldn't help myself. I couldn't believe all this. I couldn't take it all in. Where was I? Locked into a nightmare, frozen with fear and panic. Then I thought, Oh God, Caroline, not my Caroline; this can't be true.

I went into her room to find her huddled up in bed in floods of tears; she had heard my reaction. I just looked at her. I didn't know what to say or do. I couldn't grasp the reality of the situation at all. I looked at her, so ill, so hurt, so frightened. I must pull myself together, I told myself. Calm down. I had to comfort and reassure her. After all, it's just a ghastly mistake. (It was ghastly, alright, but there was no mistake.)

I tried to comfort her, but it didn't work. Rather than desperately casting around for suitable things to say there were none, only platitudes. I said nothing. I busied myself by packing an overnight bag with one or two nighties, a toothbrush and other essentials for hospital, including her favorite old gray teddy bear from childhood days. I then went to get myself organized to take her to Fairfield.

Caroline, who had been so terribly and volubly distressed, became calm, almost too calm as did I. She moved as if in a trance as we got into the car with Frank and drove from Kew to the hospital.

Caroline Hurley, new patient for admission to Ward Five, said the man into the intercom at the entrance gate. He raised the boom, and we drove slowly along the road between the old red brick buildings, jerking over the speed humps, and weaving our way past X-ray, Outpatients, Pharmacy, Pathology, all threatening new signposts in our lives, especially Caroline's, that were to become so familiar to us as we entered the time warp of the next five years. Not a single word was said.

As we drove along, I thought to myself: Fairfield. What is Fairfield? What did I know about Fairfield Infectious Diseases Hospital? All I knew then was that it was a hospital in a remote suburb that I had heard about when I was a little girl aged five; it was there that people went if they contracted infantile paralysis, or poliomyelitis, during the epidemic of 1936-37. These people, I was told, were put into iron lungs, or respirators, to have their breathing done for them in order to stay alive. I remember the 'polio victims' being wheeled along the street in long wooden prams. My mother told me that they were the ones who could breathe on their own; they could not move, though, so their real home was Fairfield. It really frightened me. And that was all I ever knew, despite having trained as a nurse at St Vincents Hospital in Melbourne in the 1950s. I don't recall that we had the option of any nursing experience at Fairfield, although we did barrier nurse patients with tuberculosis from time to time at St Vincents and also at the Austin Hospital in Ivanhoe.

By now we were in the driveway of the building which housed Ward Five. A creaking, clattering, ancient old lift with a scratched blue painted heavy door took us up to the ward. Still no words passed between us.

A kind and businesslike young nurse greeted us and ushered a tearful and stony-faced Caroline into Room Seven. It was quite an attractive room with its own little balcony overlooking the garden. Peacocks, of all things, were pecking their way among the trees on the spacious lawns. Well, thank God for a private room, I thought, even if there was no ensuite bathroom. In my confusion, I had forgotten that all patients with exotic and newly-discovered infectious diseases are nursed in isolation wards. And AIDS was a very new infectious disease. It was exotic too, in a different sense, since it was linked with an awesome fear and death.

I was dithering around, and so was Frank, not knowing what to say or do, whether to unpack Tarry's (Caroline's family name) things, or to get her into her nighty. Our behavior was making her increasingly irritated. I couldn't blame her for that. It was so awful not to be calm and competent, to be almost sick with suppressed hysteria.

The nursing staff could see our dilemma and tactfully rescued the three of us by suggesting that Frank and I return home while they admitted Tarry, attending to all the necessary formalities, arranging tests and so on. We could come back later in the day. We each kissed Caroline goodbye. It was clear that she was glad to see us go.

We drove home in an absolute daze. I don't remember how we got home, really, but as we turned into the driveway of our peaceful old home in Kew, and then sat down at the kitchen table, I just packed it in and began to cry and cry with anger, rage and self-pity. Every negative emotion that one could think of overcame me. How could this have happened to our family, to our Caroline?

Then I was seized by the thought that I must go up to Caroline's room. I wanted to see the place where I had last seen her before we took her to Fairfield. I flew up the stairs, but then stopped dead at the doorway of the second bedroom on the right. Caroline's room, the one she used to share with Kristen through their school and teenage days. Such a light and beautiful room; the best room in the house, everyone always said.

As I stepped into the room, I started to shake. I looked towards her bed and burst into tears. The small white single bed was just as she had left it that morning, a lifetime ago. The floral quilt was hanging over the side of the bed. Her pillow, all rumpled, was pushed sideways against the wall. On the floor was the soft little heap of her blue and white striped cotton nighty and the other crumpled sweat-soaked one we had changed during the night. I bent down to pick these up, thinking I must change her sheets and make everything tidy.

I couldn't do it. I felt so tired that I just lay on Caroline's bed and pulled the quilt up to my chin. Through the north-facing window, I could see the top branches of the camphor laurel tree swishing back and forth in the wind against the very blue sky. This is exactly what was happening outside that window yesterday, I thought, and the day before, and perhaps would be again tomorrow. Nothing at all had changed outside, but inside this room, this house, nothing would ever be the same again. Caroline had AIDS, and one day, I was going to lose her. I shivered with fear and cold.

As I turned my head away from the window, Tarry's Pierrot doll caught my eye. He was dangling from a shelf beside the bed, and the blue tear painted on his left cheek seemed to slip down the little white porcelain face, but it was my tears that made it look that way.

At the other end of the shelf was a zither, bought for a song by Tarry at the Camberwell market. It was propped up against her art folio with other treasures and mementos of her childhood and traveling days. I closed my eyes and inhaled the "Tarry" smells of the bed. There was the slightly acrid odor of the previous night's heavy sweats, mixed with the sweetest traces of her perfume, a slightly musky scent she had bought in Morocco. It was a type of ointment kept in a vial on her bedside table.

I must have dozed for a while, for when I opened my eyes I noticed that the sun had moved around the corner of the house and was casting dappled light through the balcony doors and onto the green carpet. I felt warm and dreamlike but then the awful reality hit me once again and I froze. Tarry had AIDS, and must surely die. This was the only truth left to me. Tarry would die but, please, not yet, not yet.

I got up, and left everything just as it was. I couldn't tidy Tarry out of that room. It was all that was left that was normal, it seemed. I closed the door and returned downstairs to the kitchen. I sat down and tried to make myself start thinking positively how was I best able to help my Tarry through the fearsome days ahead?

I really knew nothing much at all about AIDS. Before the appearance on TV of the Grim Reaper ads, I had assumed that it was confined to the male homosexual community of San Francisco, and to Uganda. Apart from some vaguely noted news reports of prostitutes who had been infected (also in Uganda, so remote and very far away from us), I didn't know even that women could catch HIV/AIDS. When the Grim Reaper ads did appear, I would watch him bowling people over at random and think, well thank God it's not happening to us. It simply never crossed my mind that it could indeed happen to our family.

As these thoughts swam around and around in my head, I had a strange vision of the Grim Reaper stalking out of the television set and heading straight for me. He wore that hideous grin of hooded death, his scythe ready to cut our lives to pieces.

I have to say that my thoughts had been solely preoccupied with myself. I hadn't even asked Frank how he was feeling, and as yet I hadn't had time to tell the other children. For all I knew, though, they may have already been told. The five of them were very close in age, and usually shared what was going on in their lives. That particular piece of information, though, Caroline might have had doubts about sharing with them. The whole thing was so totally unbelievable.

Self-doubts started creeping into my mind. Had I done the wrong thing as a mother? Had I not given her enough love? Had she had physical and emotional needs of which I had not been aware and had therefore failed to meet?

"Stop it! Stop thinking this way! You'll go mad," I said out loud to myself. Thinking this way was not going to change anything.

By the time these thoughts had been mulled over and indulged in, I had calmed down a little, had a cup of tea and started to try to piece things together rationally, carefully going over events pertaining to Tarry over the years of her early childhood.

She was 27 years of age at this time. On the day before her admission to hospital (in other words, Wednesday, October 12, which now seems a hundred years ago), we had all attended the funeral of an old aunt of mine, and after the Mass was over I noticed that Caroline seemed particularly subdued and withdrawn, not even communicating with my effusive sister and her equally chortly cousins, all girls. I also noticed that she was very, very thin.

She had been looking like this for some four to five months, not anorexic or wasted, but just so terribly thin. She had always had a fairly slight figure, but had a well-rounded bottom, in spite of being small-breasted like her sisters and myself (a physical attribute none of them thanked me for). Tarry also had stunning legs, long and shapely, and most of the time sported a very attractive suntan, which offset the dreadlocks (yes, the "dreads" were very much in vogue with our Tarry) haloing her beautiful facial contours, and brilliant, clear, well-spaced blue-green eyes. She was indeed a beauty, but now this strange thinness was draining her beauty away, and her little face looked pale, drawn and anxious. I was so puzzled by this.

I had first noticed this change in August of that year. We were on holiday at Surfers Paradise, and during that time she was having bouts of diarrhea and night sweats, as well as steady weight loss. I suggested that she see a doctor but she would have none of that, saying that she must have a bug of some sort and that she would be alright in a day or two. I let it go at that, thinking that least said, soonest mended. After all, she was an adult, and a very independent one at that. However, it was all I could do to hold my tongue when she and her sisters each bought new bathing suits in a Cavill Avenue shop. Caroline's was a child's size 14, just unbelievable, but she managed to look quite attractive in it and her appetite was good, so I let it pass.

The diarrhea, weight loss and night sweats were indicative of the onset of full-blown AIDS.

What torment Caroline must have suffered knowing this, and realizing that the time was fast approaching when she would be forced to reveal the true nature of her illness. The terror of those times for her is beyond my imagination. She had been able to keep this dread secret to herself for these past months, all the time knowing she was slowly sinking into the grip of AIDS. I will never know how Caroline endured such anguish without giving the slightest clue as to her fearful predicament. I had always thought that I could tell instinctively when something was amiss with any of my children, but this time, of all times, I suspected nothing.

Tarry did tell me much later that it was indeed worse than a nightmare. She kept trying to suppress all the horrendous fear, until it just boiled over out of her control.

When we arrived home again in Melbourne she went back to live with her friends in Brunswick, and everything seemed to be in order once more. This was in September and only four weeks of normal life were left for us, but we didn't know that at the time. Then, on the evening of October 12, at around five o'clock, Frank rang me from the Mercy Hospital, where he was the senior consultant pathologist, to tell me that Caroline was with him. He said that she was very sick indeed, and that he was sending her home to me to be looked after. She had a temperature, he explained, and needed bed-rest and the comforts of home. No other information was forthcoming.

Well, I was very happy with the prospect of caring for Caroline. I loved having the children home with me, especially one at a time. And if they were feeling poorly, I really put my heart and soul into making them comfortable and well again. Just like any other mother, I suppose. So I set about getting Caroline's room in order, fresh sheets, pillows and quilt cover; with fresh flowers by her bed; the new Vogue and Mode magazines (never to be read) and a carafe of water with a pretty glass inverted on top. When she arrived home she looked absolutely shocking. I helped her upstairs (she was so weak), undressed her, and put her to bed. Then I took her temperature. It was 41° C (106 °F). I couldn't believe it. She also had a dry cough and severe pain in her right chest wall radiating around to her back.

I was positive she had tuberculosis. I asked her whether she had been x-rayed or had given blood for testing. She didn't answer these questions very clearly, so I let her be. She was really too ill to talk much.

I tried to coax her to drink some clear chicken soup with "soldiers" (fingers of toast and Vegemite), but she couldn't swallow. So, after she had sipped a little lukewarm tea, and almost choked on two crushed

Digesic tablets, I tucked her in, kissed her and sat stroking her damp, burning forehead, until she drifted into an exhausted sleep. When I turned her light off it was 9:00 pm.

By this time Frank had arrived home. We were having a drink before dinner when I voiced my fears about the possibility of Caroline having TB. How could she have got it, why wasn't she having the appropriate tests, and what did he make of all this?

Frank, hesitating a little, said that she definitely had a serious illness, but we were not to worry about it now. It would all be sorted out the next day. I could see there was no point in questioning Frank any further, so after dinner we went up to bed. I was very tired, but too anxious and worried to sleep. It must have been extremely hard for Frank, for he already knew the truth: Caroline had told him that afternoon at the Mercy, and together they had tried to sort out the best way of telling me. But there was no easy way.

I heard Caroline stirring during the night and went into her room to find her absolutely saturated in a sweat-soaked bed. I helped her take a quick shower, remade her bed and put a clean nighty over her head. I sat with her, stroking her head again, until she seemed to sleep.

It was definitely TB. No sleep for me for many nights to come, for that was the beginning of the nightmare. Tests at Fairfield had already identified a special strain of TB – AIDS-related TB.

CHAPTER 2

❧

TRANQUIL SEAS RECALLED

Well, the unthinkable had actually happened. AIDS had struck where least expected – a heterosexual daughter of a normal Catholic middle-class family living in Kew, Melbourne, Australia. Ours was a united and happy family, well-educated, comfortably housed, and above all, very well loved and cherished. Each and every one of our four daughters and only son were wonderful, soundly adjusted, steady young adults, with good jobs. They were each making a fair contribution to home and country, and showed the fulfillment of the promise that had been there from the very beginning of our marriage.

Our wedding day was on January 10, 1959. It was a fiercely hot midsummer's day, 41°C (106°F), but I hardly noticed the heat as my sister Maria and the two bridesmaids helped me into my long white dress. I was just twenty-one, and was so excited, sick with nerves, and, at that time, terribly thin. I was madly in love and dying to marry Frank.

The girls attached the veil to my short fair hair and I thought I was Christmas. I am pleased to say that Frank did, too. He stood at the top of the aisle in the chapel and watched me approach, clinging to my father's arm. I held Frank's gaze as I walked slowly towards him and I knew I would always be loved and safe. And I always have been.

Once married, we were very anxious to have children. This was mainly because of the difference in our ages. Frank is 17 years older than I, so we were delighted when Kristen was born in November of that year. She was followed 14 months later by Caroline, in another 14 months Jamie arrived, 14 months later Margie then another 17 months and Dominique was born.

We were becoming rather worried as to just how many more children I would produce. Contraception was not an option for us at the time; we were practicing Catholics, and the Church forbade any form of artificial child prevention. Luckily, my reproductive organs went on strike, so to speak, and I had no more pregnancies after that. Of course, five children in as many years was not considered unusual in those times, especially in Catholic families. Some couples we knew had 12 children. They were amazing how they managed.

We found our five quite enough to handle. It was hard work trying to give each one their fair share of quality time and attention. Those baby days were wonderful, though, as well as very busy, and Frank was always a great help, in spite of his long days in the pathology departments of the hospitals in which he worked.

Those five children were very different little people, in appearance and personalities.

Kristen, who was shy, studious and quiet, had quite a witty personality, which took many years to manifest itself fully. For a long time she seemed to be buried under the weight of her more outgoing and exuberant siblings.

Caroline was anything but quiet, at least on the home front. She was a very pretty child with a hearty, boisterous laugh. She was the pivot of family fun and affection. She also had quite a fiery temper, which often triggered off the usual family fights and arguments. Caroline was our "comic strip." From quite an early age, she possessed an infectious gaiety. I remember her witticisms as quite preposterous, sometimes startling and often unintentional.

One night, when Tarry was eight, we were having roast leg of pork for someone's birthday dinner. Tarry asked, "What kind of a bird is a pork?" She had only ever seen chicken served up with legs before. We all fell about with laughter as Frank explained what a "pork" really was.

Other queries like "What time is the six o'clock news?" were remembered with affection by all of us, and she happily stood up to the laughter and teasing they aroused. Even at this age Tarry's personality was developing and becoming quite strikingly obvious. When she evoked laughter in the family or with friends, there was no element of scorn, and when she provoked teasing, no trace of malice. Spontaneity was second nature to her and her innate simplicity mirrored her sincerity. In later years these features of her character probably accounted for her capacity to form close and lasting friendships with little effort.

As a young adult Tarry was not above practicing a degree of deceit at times (she was no paragon), but she never mastered the art. In fact, she was a complete duffer. I can honestly say that as a young girl, as a teenager and also as a young adult (even in her darkest hours), Tarry remained a very potent force in the binding love that united our family. In the years to come she was to become in many ways its linchpin.

Kristen and Tarry's bedroom here at Kew opened onto a balcony which runs across the front of the house upstairs. Pigeons had occupied that balcony and its wide gray cement-rendered ledge since time immemorial. There they had had free reign to build their nests, copulate, procreate and defecate. There were mountains of pigeon poo along the full length of that balcony. If those droppings could have found a market, another of Melbourne's Nauru house could have been built on the proceeds.

These pigeons drove us crazy with their mess and their incessant noise "gorrorp, gorrorp, gorrorp" both day and night, if disturbed. Even when Tarry went running out on the balcony, crunching over the droppings in her pajamas, yelling "gorrorp" right back at them, they would just sit there and continue. They were completely unafraid. It was hilarious to watch, but in the end something had to be done to remove them. The pest controllers were called in. Don't kill the "gorrorps," Tarry pleaded.

Drug-impregnated bird seed was scattered along the balcony and the roof. The pigeons ate this seed and, one by one, flew away. They would never return to Tarry's balcony, for their homing instinct had been destroyed by the bird seed. All pigeons anywhere are now called "gorrorps" thanks to Tarry.

Magpies were renamed "gorkelorkels" after their musical serenades on the front lawn in the spring and summer. Tarry would call to them "gorkelorkel" and they would cock their heads with curiosity and cautiously quick-step to her for little bits of bread. It was a wonderful sight.

Our grandchildren, who are just beginning to talk, now respond to "gorrorp" and "gorkelorkel" and can identify the birds by those names. Another little legacy from their Aunt Caroline, whom they never knew, but will always remember.

Tarry was said to have my personality. I am very happy about that, for she was great fun, bossy, level-headed, practical, occasionally bad-tempered, adventurous, generous, sensitive and kind. So if I am like that, I am very pleased indeed. I have written more about Tarry, because this is part of her completed story. The others still have their lives to lead and their stories will unfold as the years roll by.

Jamie, the only boy, was right in the middle of the four girls. But that didn't bother him at all. He was, and still is, good to his sisters, although he wasn't averse to giving Margie the occasional swift kick, and even tipped her out of her pram when she was tiny. His life was full of sport, study, surfboards, guitars, both classical and electric, golf clubs and a host of friends.

Margie was sweet and gentle, funny, clever and very lovable, and she remains so today. When little, though, she used to be a colossal whiner if she felt she was being swamped by the family circus. She was a very courteous child and so kind, and so very little that nappies would dangle round her ankles as she toddled around at nine months of age. Margie has proved to be my rod and my staff and my mentor. If this makes her appear to be the family favorite, this is not so, for each is special in their own way.

Dominique, the baby, spent most of her time keeping up with the others. Highly competitive, argumentative and gifted, it was not until she was well into her twenties that she knew where those gifts lay. She is now a talented furniture maker.

Although each was quite unique and very special, as a young mother I tended to lump the children all in together. I would only glimpse or be aware of their individuality when time or circumstance permitted. This tendency to clock watch has always been with me, a need to get things done. One fairly astonishing way in which I would try to do this was the manner in which I fed them "brekky." I would have one large bowl of cornflakes and fruit, and one spoon. I would sit on one side of the kitchen table, and have the children all lined up in a row on the other side, bibs on, like little birds. I would give them a spoonful each, one after the other. They actually found this great fun, but I don't know where that would put me as a mother on the scale of one to ten in this day and age.

So perhaps they did have to fight for individual attention, more than children in better-spaced families. Well, no family is perfect, I suppose. In spite of all this, I really felt the children and I had a great relationship. There was definitely no shortage of love and demonstrative affection.

The children were all very different, of course. They endured various scrapes in and out of school, had many good friends, plenty of fun, ups and downs, and we all enjoyed everything together. Among the worst incidents I knew of included the time Jamie, who is now a doctor, was caught smoking outside the school gates. Dominique, too, was caught smoking behind the lavatories at school.

Margie distinguished herself by giving her classmates a demonstration, in the classroom, of wading through the trees of adolescence while, unknown to our Margie, the religious knowledge teacher looked on. Margie was suspended from that class for three weeks. She is now a solicitor, and a good one at that. Kristen, a hospital scientist, didn't seem to get into trouble, being a little less extroverted than her siblings.

Tarry was different again. At home she was always bright and bubbly, but at school she had trouble settling in right from her kindergarten days. She was very frightened of the nun in charge of the "kinder," and was not the only little one in that position. The poor nun had been running the "kinder" for many, many years — far too long. She was much too old for the job, and her old-fashioned severity frightened and stultified the behavior of the more timid "littlies," one of whom was our Tarry.

During her late junior school days, Tarry also suffered a long period of peer group taunting (about what I don't know). She said little or nothing about this, but when it all came to light, there were terrible scenes, and mortified girls penned letters of apology not only to Tarry, but to Frank and me as well. She never forgot that time, but she did get over it. Strangely enough, it was those very trouble-makers who in later years were to form the nucleus of Tarry's staunchest supporters, the "card girls." Their unconditional care and love stayed with Tarry all through her life.

As Tarry grew older, things seemed to improve for her. She was studying graphic art, making new friends and becoming more confident and jolly as her beauty of mind and body developed.

Now, though, this happy family of five children, each of whom had cavorted and studied their way through their years of school and tertiary education with some good measure of success, was faced by catastrophe. The all too real world had caught up with them and they now faced a stark and horrible truth – the eventual and almost certain death of their beloved sister and friend, their pal Caroline.

Chapter 3

༈

The Clouds Gather

Every detail of the early morning of Thursday, October 13, 1988, is still vivid in my mind. The events of the late afternoon and evening have become, with the passage of time, and no doubt due to the shock we had experienced, much less clear in my mind and in Frank's.

I do remember Caroline begging us not to tell anyone about her having AIDS because of the stigma associated with the disease. She included her brother and sisters in this. We were to tell them and anyone else who asked why she was in Fairfield Hospital that she had come down with tuberculosis – "normal" TB of course. At that time, a number of cases had been reported, so this explanation would not seem too far-fetched.

However, it seemed to us impossible and impractical not to tell the children the truth. The same evening after dinner, I told Dominique. She was terribly shocked, and grieved, but her sole concern was for Tarry. Frank told Margie and she reacted in the same way. I was so moved by their expressions of genuine love and concern for their beloved big sister and, at the same time, struggling valiantly to deal with the enormous belting blows of shock raining down on them.

Frank told Jamie and Kristen within the next 24 hours and they too accepted the dreadful news in such a loving and supportive way that, when over the course of the next few days, Tarry realized they knew the truth, she did not object. She made no further specific requests regarding her HIV/AIDS status, but we knew that she was desperate not to have the news spread. Any enquiries about where and how she was were really answered quite truthfully, as she did have TB.

After all this, I was so panicked that I actually had the temerity to ask them all to undergo HIV testing. After all, if Caroline could and did succumb to it, couldn't they also be infected? It was a terrible thing to ask of them, but I know they understood my motive. I never mentioned it again, so I have never found out if they actually did have the test. Anyway, the ensuing years have shown that they did not have AIDS.

What had prompted me to make this request was an article I had read in a newspaper about a mother in England who had lost her entire family of six children to AIDS, and I thought, My God, will this happen to us as well?

Although this did not happen, the children were all forced to adjust to the fact that Caroline and Fairfield would very likely become the focal point of our lives as parents from now until whenever (if only we could have thought "if ever") she died. It was going to be very hard to give each one a fair go as the years went by.

At the same time, some sort of normal routine had to be maintained in our respective households. Caroline insisted on this. She was desperate not to create waves , as she put it. After all, they were adults now and had their lives to live, careers to establish, studies to do, and would in the future have their own families to care for.

Kristen, the eldest, had married in June of 1988, which, Caroline later told me, is why she had not said anything about her illness, in case she spoiled her sister's wedding, at which she was chief bridesmaid. I believed her, and admired her bravery.

I was the one who had the most difficulty in adapting to the situation. I was all over the place. During Caroline's first two weeks in hospital, I would be calmly conducting the family orchestra at home one minute, and then the next, when I was by myself, I would be falling apart with fear, grief and pain. The customary evening brandy and soda, followed by wine with dinner, did nothing to relieve this. In fact, it only made things worse – I felt weepy and nauseated. Eventually, though, I did become accustomed to the daily visits to Caroline, who was now tolerating naso-gastric feeding of Ensure Plus, and was taking anti-tubercular medication plus antibiotics.

Other things, however, were not so easy to get used to nor should they have been. One day on this first hospital visit, Caroline was being taken by ambulance to the Sacred Heart Hospital in Moreland for a CAT scan. She was terribly hurt by a remark concerning her that was made by a nurse assisting the ambulance man: "Watch out for this one. She's got AIDS."

I was absolutely horrified when she told me. I hadn't dreamed of prejudice where Caroline was concerned. She became rather cynical about this incident, although I am pleased to say that it was an isolated event. And our deep love and concern for her would negate all that, as it would other anxieties that distressed her. Our darling Caroline thought she had disgraced the family by getting AIDS. What a load of rubbish. How could we think such a thing? The fact that AIDS is sex-related was irrelevant. So many young people were sexually active, Catholic or otherwise, and it was just a cruel blow of fate to collect AIDS along the way.

Initially I had not thought it wise to ask Caroline how she had become infected. It was bad enough for her having us know that she was. However, some time later Caroline confided in me that she had believed that taking the contraceptive pill would prevent AIDS. Clearly ignorance was all around us. She told me that she had had a relationship with a bisexual young man in 1982. She had not known that he was bisexual at that time but at a Christmas party in December 1987 she had heard him being discussed. The fact that he was HIV positive had come to light. Although many years had passed since she had seen him, she had gone to the Sexually Transmitted Diseases (STD) clinic and, to her horror, was tested positive.

I suggested killing him there and then, but Caroline said not to worry as he was already dead. That was not true, as I discovered much later. At the time, though, that story was quite acceptable to us. It was one less thing to concern us. I thought it considerate of Caroline to have dealt with things that way.

Until Caroline's visit to the STD clinic and my subsequent visit there to collect some pamphlets outlining care of patients with AIDS at home (that, too was an awful ordeal), I had thought STD was an inter-state phone call or Doctor of Sacred Theology, the title of one of my more learned priest friends. SIDA, the European acronym for AIDS, I had thought was a type of small Italian car, such was my ignorance at that time.

But I was learning many new things as each day passed. Caroline was terribly afraid that she was going to die very soon. Well, any time is too soon – be it five years or five minutes – but she was looking at the short term with a great deal of fear. I remember holding her close to me for hours one night in Room Seven at Fairfield. I rocked her gently like a baby, crooning softly to her and promising her that she would not die. No way would I let my Caroline die not if I could help it.

On my birthday, October 19, I missed her presence so much. We had always been great birthday celebrators, and would have family dinners with friends along as well. But this year there was this awful gap at the table. I wondered if Tarry would ever celebrate any more birthdays with us, and yes, I started to cry again.

I simply had to stop feeling sorry for myself, I decided. I had to get on with living and not make family and friends uncomfortable around me. In some ways, however, I made them more uncomfortable, with false, shrieking, brittle chatter. I had always had a reputation for being the so-called life of the party, but now it had a hollow ring to it and was driving the family mad.

I came to realize the truth of this when I accidentally came across a letter written to Tarry by one of her sisters. It had not been given to her, it seemed, and was just lying in the bottom of a drawer, where I discovered it as I was tidying up. Part of the contents of the letter were apologies to Tarry for Mum's irritating behavior, so there must have been some discussion between them.

I took good notice of this and endeavored to regain a more natural and composed approach to what was happening. It was an almost impossible task, but it did help to create a more stable atmosphere when I simmered down.

My sister was marvelous. She made pretty nighties and pillow cases for Tarry and kept her laughing with funny stories, cards and lots of flowers. There was an atmosphere of humor, homeliness, warmth and security taking over sterile little room number Seven in Ward Five.

Frank went to great trouble to buy some really comfortable fluffy sheepskin slippers for Tarry's very thin, weak cold feet. They were pink, and when he gave them to her, Tarry's face lit up and she hugged them to her as she expressed her joy and thanks to her dad. She kept them with her through the ensuing years. A small thing perhaps, but a huge triumph for Frank, to have been able to provide a special comfort for her, when he could not provide a cure.

For nearly two years now, Tarry had had a steady boyfriend, and they seemed to be very much in love. He was a strange young man, tall and handsome. He proposed marriage to Tarry while she was in hospital, and her joy was truly wondrous to behold, even though she and everyone else was cruelly aware that she would never marry, and would never have the children I knew she longed for one day. She proudly wore a little pearl and gold ring that she was given as a sign of their betrothal. Family and friends showered them with congratulatory gifts, flowers, and other expressions of their joy for them.

Frank and I, with the rest of the family, made a pretence of happiness and joy for Tarry, but we felt that the whole thing was something of a charade. We were so worried about her condition that we were more than happy for any occurrence that would bring smiles to her anxious little face. This betrothal, in fact, came to nothing. He was to prove a great source of trouble and anxiety over the years, and as a result I came to dislike him intensely in the end, but I suppose they were happy with each other at times.

He seemed to have no close friends and was apparently not very close to his family. He could give the impression of being very knowledgeable and was full of theories and ambitious plans. However, he had no specific qualifications and no regular work. He gave the impression that the world owed him a living. Alcohol was a major problem and, at Kristen's wedding in June 1988, he had to be forcibly evicted from the reception, having got so drunk that he was attacking one or two of the male guests. In time we came to learn that he had HIV.

His father, however, was quite a remarkable man. He was marvelous with Tarry. He really loved and admired her, and would sit for hours by her hospital bed, encouraging her and strengthening her will to live. I was very grateful to him, although we were never to know each other well. That didn't matter. He helped Tarry when she needed help, that was enough for me.

After two weeks in Fairfield, Caroline was well enough to come home to Kew, which she did on October 26, complete with naso-gastric feeding tube, many cans of Ensure Plus and a bottle of Coca-Cola with a large syringe but no needle. These last two items were to be used if the tube became blocked with dried food and debris. The Coke acted as a solvent in the blocked naso-gastric tube. And of course, the tube did block, especially at night. There were several occasions during which I would draw up 10 milliliters of Coke and squirt it down the tube, so that Tarry had to endure a blast of Coca-Cola into her tummy. We even managed to laugh about it, she and I, as we worked by torchlight to unblock the wretched tube.

She also brought home with her an outpatient's appointment card which listed all her medications and the times they were to be taken. The huge paper bag full of pills was eventually replaced by a box with compartments for days of the week and times, which made the pill-taking procedure much easier. There were so many of them and they had to be crushed up with a mortar and pestle, mixed with water and squirted down the feeding tube.

As I sat down to read the card, I noticed the signature of the resident medical officer. He had a German name, which when translated into English meant "God's child." I remember wondering how many of God's children with HIV/AIDS he had seen and treated, and would eventually see off to God. It was a strange feeling.

Tarry was still very weak, but her mood was brighter, and she was able to tolerate small amounts of soft food by mouth – a source of great joy to me as I riffled through the pages of an old "invalid cookery" book, seeking something new and appetizing to prepare for her. Actually most of the recipes were revolting, but could be modified using modern ingredients.

It was now late October, just a little over two weeks since the dreadful news had broken.

Only people who have lived in Melbourne fully understand the significance of the forthcoming first Tuesday in November. This is Melbourne Cup day, the focal point of a whole week of wonderful racing, parties and entertainment – highlighted by the huge influx of overseas visitors and associated social events. Frank and I had always been involved wholeheartedly in all of this since the early days of our married life. We had owned and raced horses and the children had always enjoyed and appreciated Frank's love of the thoroughbred.

But all this vanished in the wink of an eye now that our beloved daughter had AIDS. Tarry and I had heated discussions about Cup Week. She insisted that we go and keep up pretenses. I said, "no way." The very thought of it all made me feel really sick. Such trivial frivolity had no further place in our lives, I thought. Frank was inclined to agree with Caroline's idea in order to keep curious questioners at bay: if we kept our race-week commitments then her secret would remain safe. Tarry was adamant that we carry on as usual.

We were both being quite irrational. Our world was crashing down around us, and I was dazed and dithery. Stupidly, I went ahead with some of the planned Cup Week activities for which I would pay with a huge draining of my physical and emotional resources. On Friday, Derby eve, I had my hair done. When I came home from the hairdresser, I noticed that Tarry was becoming quite ill again. I took her temperature. It was 40°C (104°F). She had developed a blotchy, itching rash on her arms and the pain in her chest had returned. She was very distressed and frightened, and so was I. The doctor, however, was unable to come until the Saturday morning.

By the morning, it was quite obvious that I would not be going to the Derby. Tarry was much worse. The rash had spread over her entire body and was just unbearable. She was beside herself with the terrible itching and pain and nausea. Margie came over to Kew to help me soothe Tarry while we waited for the doctor to arrive.

We helped Tarry into a warm bath, having added sodium bicarbonate to the water in an effort to relieve her unbearable itching. This used to be good in the old days when the children caught chicken pox, the five of them one after the other. Unfortunately it was not at all effective for Tarry – if anything, it aggravated the symptoms this time. Margie dabbed Tarry's tormented body dry, whispering soothing words of quiet comfort to her as she did so. It was a very moving scene for anyone to witness, with the tears now flowing down our faces.

We had all decided that it would be best for Frank to leave Margie and me to look after Tarry, and go to the Derby with our Sydney friends, who had always shared this week with us. Off they went, and soon after, the doctor from the STD clinic arrived. She was a lovely young woman whom Tarry knew, liked and trusted.

Apparently, Tarry was having a severe reaction to one of the anti-tubercular medications. For the past ten days or so she had been taking a very high dosage of it. The doctor ordered the appropriate antidote and ointment, and reduced the dosage of the oral medication. As soon as we had the appropriate medication, Margie ever so gently applied the ointment, and the medication gradually took effect, allowing the angry itchy, blotchy rash to disappear.

By the next day, Sunday, October 30, Tarry was feeling much better. She insisted that Frank and I go to a luncheon party organized by some enthusiastic racing friends. I really couldn't have thought of anything worse, but we went along.

For the next two days Tarry's condition was quite good, so I made the huge effort of going out to the Melbourne Cup on the first Tuesday in November. I was dressed to kill, but actually looked like death. We piled the usual picnic fare into the boot of the car and drove out to Flemington.

It was a disaster. I sat in the car park sobbing all day. I hated every minute of the long hours out there. I wanted to come home to Tarry, which we eventually did. Thank God the Melbourne Cup was over at last for another year. I have never really enjoyed the races since that day. During the day it gradually became apparent to those around us that Frank and I were not our usual selves. Our closest friends were sufficiently sensitive to see through our pretense and by the end of the day, we had no option but to confide in two or three couples. These trusted friends did not betray our confidence and each of them was very fond of Caroline.

Although outwardly things were more normal, the pain in Tarry's chest was now becoming more severe. Her temperature was swinging up and down each day. I made an appointment for her in outpatients at Fairfield on Friday, November 4. Tarry would need to have some sort of medicated inhalation, followed by yet another CAT scan at Moreland. This time, I would take her. No prejudiced paramedics were going to get within cooee of my daughter ever again. Not if I could help it.

We drove first to Fairfield, where we parked the car and followed the signs along the glassed-in red-brick verandas to the day center. This was a truly horrifying experience. I have never before or since seen any-thing to equal the scene we beheld. Tarry had turned as white as a sheet, and my heart started missing beats then thumped rapidly. For there in this fairly small room were massed together what seemed like hundreds of men in various stages of AIDS illnesses. They sat in wheel chairs, armchairs, wooden benches, all with blood transfusions dripping into their thin and blotchy arms. Some had strange disfiguring marks on their faces. It was horrendous.

Tarry and I were speechless with shock. I felt a rising terror that Tarry would have to suffer in the same way as these young men were suffering. I thought that at any moment I was going to be sick, and Tarry felt the same way. Luckily, though, we weren't.

To make matters worse, I looked across the room and there was a nun with whom I had once nursed sitting beside one of the young men. She was the only other female in this room. I thought, screaming inside myself, "Don't, please, please, please, dear God, don't let her see me. Don't recognize me, look away from me!" She did see me, but she also showed no sign of knowing me, which was lucky, as Tarry was still averse to letting outsiders know of her condition.

The room resembled a miniature battlefield. As long as I live, the memory of it will remain fixed in my brain. It was a terrible intro-duction to the cruel reality of AIDS, a reality which, as the years went on, I would come to know very well. My awareness and understanding of what AIDS does to its victims "bodies and minds" would come to know no bounds. My compassion for all those infected people would grow from small beginnings in direct proportion to my hatred of the virus itself.

I approached the doctor sitting at a small table in the center of this room and introduced Tarry and myself to him. I begged him to let us be in a room by ourselves, even if it was a broom cupboard. Tarry and I were both close to tears, but for once I managed to control myself. We were finally ushered into the requested room, marginally bigger than a broom cupboard, where Tarry's treatment would be carried out. The doctor said we would need the assistance of a nurse. I told him I was a nurse and if he explained what was required I would manage it, and I did.

Until that moment Tarry and I had thought that Pentamidine was another AIDS-Related Condition (ARC), which would be treated by PCP. In fact, PCP was the illness, Pneumocystic Carinii Pneumonia, that the doctors were trying to prevent Tarry from acquiring, through the use of a Pentamidine spray, which was inhaled into the lungs via an oxygen cylinder. So we really had got things back to front, in all the confusion.

The doctor sat Tarry down and connected the inhalation, which was to be used for approximately 30 minutes, during which time I was to monitor her blood pressure. I had been warned that it could drop to a very low level, and this is in fact what happened. I was very glad I had been told what to expect or I might have thought that Tarry was about to die. As it was, I nearly died of fright myself.

After resting for some time after this treatment, Tarry felt well enough to walk back to the car, where we sat with the Melways road map trying to work out how to get to the Sacred Heart Hospital in Moreland. Tarry was absolutely wonderful. She carefully navigated me along Heidelberg Road and cross-country to Moreland. I was a wreck and she had the giggles. How I loved my Tarry.

I had Frank's hospital car park sticker, which I thought I would use to save looking for a park in the nearby streets. I drove into the doctors' car park and immediately backed into another doctor's car. I couldn't believe it. No damage was done, though, and by this time Tarry and I were hysterical with laughter. Our emotions were in a state of chaos.

The laughter fell silent as we entered the door of the CAT scan department. No warm greetings there. Tarry was just another patient on the assembly line, and I was ignored completely. To be fair, the staff were quite obviously run off their feet. Tarry didn't seem to mind, so neither did I. How we got through all these events together without falling apart was a miracle. It was mainly due to Tarry's common sense, bravery and sense of humor. She simply amazed me.

When we arrived home at Kew, Tarry said she felt alright, and that she would like to return to her friends in Brunswick for that weekend, maybe even longer. I was very doubtful about this, but she was the best judge of how she felt, and altogether it seemed a good idea to have a break from each other and the hospital circuit for a while.

It turned out to be a very good idea indeed. It gave me the opportunity to get some order into the household again. Christmas was approaching and I always cooked the puddings during the week after Cup week. I shopped for the ingredients, soaked the fruit, mixed the mixture, divided it between the pudding bowls, forgot to add the flour, got the mixture out again, mixed in the flour, then put everything back into the bowls, along with a few silver coins from pre-decimal currency days. I covered the bowls with foil and string, and away those puddings bubbled and cooked. I felt wonderful. The house was cleaned, the ironing and shopping was done, and some decent meals were able to be presented for nearly a whole week.

With things now more settled, I suggested to Tarry that we have a few days together at Portsea, on the Mornington Peninsula, at our little beach house. She was feeling much better and happily agreed to this. So on Friday, November 11, on a really lovely afternoon, we drove there together. We planned to meet up with one of Tarry's friends who lived near Portsea at Rye. We would have a picnic together on Portsea back beach, at London Bridge – an enormous rocky arch situated on the shoreline at the Point Nepean end of the huge surfing beach.

We also hoped to spend some time at Point King. This is a small and beautiful stretch of sandy bayside beach located between Portsea and Sorrento. It is quite secluded, and dotted along the edge of the teatree between the cliff and sand are little white beach boxes. Two boat jetties that project out from this little cove provide a safe boundary for children playing in and out of the water.

Along with many other families with young children, our family had spent every summer beach day there for nearly 25 years. Each year the same families would occupy the same patch of beach. There was quite a territorial feel about this. Our position was known as Vatican City , because each of the six or so families who gathered there was predominantly Catholic, and between us all we had about 30 children.

Those were our truly happy times – the long hot summer days at Point King. The children, all healthy, strong and exuberant, played so happily together, swimming, building sand castles, snorkeling, catching leatherjackets in fishing nets, and sometimes rowing little dinghies under strict parental supervision. Lunch was bread rolls, a banana and bottled water or fruit juice.

The mums, and sometimes dads, if they were not working back in town, all sat on little beach seats under beach umbrellas, and would keep a sharp eye on our own and each others children as we chatted about nothing much or nothing very serious. We were so comfortable in each others company, as were the children. At the end of each day we would reluctantly organize the gathering up of thongs, T-shirts and towels and shepherd tired and often grizzling young ones up the steep path back to the family cars. The kids always used to yell affectionate goodbyes to each other, with promises to meet up the next day, same beach, same time. It was just wonderful.

Tarry would often take the hand of a weary little one or carry them up the path to spare small, tired legs from being scratched by the box thorn bushes and teatree which lined the narrow stony path. When we were all piled into the car, she would strike up a singsong. All the family joined in, shouting the same silly ditty every day, with all windows wound down.

We'll drink a drink a drink
To Lily the Pink the Pink the Pink,
The savior of the Human Ra-a-ace!
She invented medicinal compound
Most efficacious in every case.*

I can still hear them singing this, as clearly now as I did in those lovely cruisy, carefree days, and I weep for those days long gone. Foolishly I wish Lily the Pink could have dreamed up a medicinal compound for AIDS.

All the children loved Point King and used to dream about taking their own children there one day. Most of them do just that, but the most enthusiastic dreamer was the very one who missed out. Tarry and I did visit there from time to time, though, when she was well enough to negotiate that steep path. Towards the end of her life, when she could

---

* From "Lily the Pink" by Gorman, McGear, McGough. Copyright © 1968 by Noel Gay Music Co. Ltd. Reproduced by permission of Campbell Connelly (Australia) Pty Ltd.

no longer walk unaided, her father carried her down to Point King for one last lingering look. It nearly broke Frank's heart. I was not with them on that occasion. It was a precious moment shared by father and daughter only a few weeks before Tarry was to die.

As it turned out, I didn't get to spend time with Tarry at Point King on this particular occasion either. Soon after our arrival at Portsea Tarry began to feel unwell. The pain in her chest was back, her temperature was up again, and she was also quite lethargic. A panicky feeling started to shiver in my chest. I rang Jamie, our son, by then a doctor, and I asked him what I should do. He calmly suggested that I take Tarry into the nearest hospital for a chest X-ray.

I did this, and nothing more sinister than usual turned up. I don't think I mentioned AIDS at the hospital, probably for fear of any reactions of prejudice among the staff. I was really sensitive about this, much more so than Tarry.

Things settled down again, the pain eased, and Tarry was able to visit her friend, but it was too cold at London Bridge for a picnic during our stay. We came back to Melbourne on Wednesday, November 16, and Tarry once more returned to Brunswick.

Illness struck her again on the following Sunday. Swollen glands and a raging fever meant going back to Fairfield for more blood tests and X-rays. The situation was to remain like this for some time – into Fairfield for a few days, home again. Back to Fairfield. On and on and on it went, with Tarry becoming more and more depressed and me not knowing which way to turn.

On November 28, Kristen's birthday, Caroline came home feeling well enough to join in the birthday dinner, but although her appetite was good, she was still deeply depressed. On November 30, Caroline was back at Fairfield yet again. This occasion, though, would be quite a momentous one, and a fearful one also. For on this day Caroline was to begin her first actual treatment for the AIDS virus, with the drug AZT. It was a very big step into the unknown, for there was little to go on as to the effectiveness of this drug. At the time, AZT was thought to stave off invasion of life-threatening illnesses in both males and females.

I don't know what the side effects were supposed to be, but as far as I could see, Caroline tolerated AZT very well, apart from a fairly minimal hair loss. The dreadlocks she had once worn had long since been detached from her head.

After another dose of Pentamidine, which was later changed to Dapsone tablets to spare Caroline the discomfort of the inhalation, her discharge was arranged. An outpatients appointment was made so that she could be reviewed on December 14. Caroline asked me never to visit OP with her again, and I didn't. She valued her independence and she felt sure she would cope better without me around. I was grateful for that. She knew that I would be there by her side if she needed me.

Christmas was now really looming up and things were looking good again. I did all the Christmas shopping in one day. Something for everyone. I felt marvelous. I love shopping; I call it "retail" therapy. When everything is going well, or badly, there's nothing to equal pottering around the shops with the credit card tap-tapping to get out of the purse.

I even managed to play a bit of golf with Frank. I had recently been accepted as a member of one of the golf clubs in Kew. Although I had no golfing prowess, in spite of lessons from patient professionals, when able to enjoy them the exercise and fresh air were great. Frank and I would use this time to try to relax a little and also to discuss Tarry's progress, as progress it mostly was those days, although there was plenty of drama sandwiched in between each positive step.

I also squeezed in a two-day trip to Sydney, to stay with another close friend. When I came home, though, Tarry was in hospital again. She was allowed home for the night on Christmas Eve, and watched me set the table with the best silver and glasses. She put Christmas crackers on everyone's place mat and then sat with me in the kitchen while I prepared the vegetables, glazed the ham, stuffed the turkey, and did other little trimmings for Christmas dinner.

We wrapped presents together. Her slender hands, with their long, beautiful fingers, trembled with fatigue as she tried to tie the ribbons, so she stopped that and hung a few baubles on the Christmas tree instead. With all jobs completed, it was very peaceful and Christmassy, but Tarry was exhausted, so I tucked her into bed quite early. I slipped into bed beside her and we discussed how to take care of her health properly without her feeling too smothered by me. Although she was still depressed and angry about her illness, she was in fact adjusting to the inevitable that she was stuck with things as they were at least as regards her health.

She wanted to live her life as normally as possible as soon as she could. This was her short-term goal and she was working hard to achieve it. We agreed that she could live at Brunswick with her boyfriend and friends in their rather ramshackle, but unprejudiced, home while she was feeling well, but she must return home to me if she became ill. She had to promise to do this. This arrangement was successful for quite some time and took the pressure off her, and off family and friends as well.

Christmas Day 1988 was really a great success, even though Tarry was unable to tolerate much of the food. She was determined to manage a little Chrissy pud and brandy sauce, though, and she did. Meanwhile it was still the Ensure Plus naso-gastric tube feeding that was successfully providing her with all the nourishment she required.

Kristen had given Tarry a beautiful white cane rocking chair, well padded with cushions and colorful pillows, and she rocked back and forth in her nighty and new dressing gown, a very posh one of thick toweling that was Margie's gift to her. And of course, Tarry was wearing Frank's fluffy pink slippers. She loved his gift to her so much. Friends called in and everyone was quite relaxed, and not too solicitous of Tarry, for which she was very grateful.

It was back to Fairfield after that, to stay there until the following week. New Year's Eve passed by quietly enough, ushering in the terrible year of 1989; more terrible for me, it seemed, than for Tarry, if that could be possible.

Tarry had again begun to show some improvement – actually, a great deal of improvement would be closer to the truth. She began to take more and more food orally. However, the tube had to stay in place. She would counter any questions about this tube by saying, "The tube is in because I can't eat properly. I have an ulcer in my gullet." Everyone accepted that, and out she went sailing, swimming, cycling, walking along her favorite Portsea back beach to London Bridge. In short, she did everything her family and friends did, except perhaps for shorter periods and with the naso-gastric tube as her talisman. (This tube is quite long and narrow. It is inserted into the patient's nostril, goes up the bridge of the nose, down the patient's chest in line with the breast bone, and then into the stomach.)

It was marvelous to see her lovely little face filled out, shiny clear eyes, all smiles again, and her body rounding out once more. Those shapely legs, tanned anew, were being flashed around in new denim shorts, with a navy and white striped polo shirt worn on top. It was very attractive and was sloppy enough to disguise the thinness of her chest wall and upper arms, which worried her for a while.

Tarry's hair was almost completely gray as it grew back. The Hurley side of the family all tend towards premature grayness, but our Tarry would have none of that so she bought a rich brown hair coloring agent and after messing up the bathroom totally, emerged looking gorgeous, with brand new hair. We all admired and applauded her. Her energy levels and strength were increasing day by day. Her general appearance was that of a very well person.

Tarry's birthday occurs on January 23, and this year she was turning twenty-eight. What a party we had for her at Portsea. It was absolutely fantastic. A number of her friends came to celebrate and stay with us. They were still marveling at Caroline's acceptance of her illness and her resilience, and also at her gutsy manner in fighting this disease.

She was not going to give in without a huge battle. The haunted look of fear and hopelessness had left those lovely eyes, and she was ready to take on the world. Well, she sure took on her birthday party, leaving the rest of us limp in a corner as she danced on.

The highlight of the evening was the dinner cooked by Dominique. She prepared the most wonderful bouillabaisse, Tarry's favorite, and so easy to eat. It was brim full of beautiful, fresh seafood – crayfish, mussels, scallops, prawns, all cooked in a delicious homemade fish stock, and served in a huge black enamel pot with lots of crusty homemade bread. Dominique is a superb cook and she drew upon all her culinary expertise to put this together for her sister. My contribution was an Italian dessert, tira-mi-su, surrounded by fresh berries, and a red candle on top for presentation as a birthday cake. We all sang, "For she's a jolly good lassie," because our Tarry was indeed a jolly good lassie.

Tarry continued to improve. She swallowed all her myriad multi-colored pills, along with the blue and white AZT capsules, each with a little galloping horse printed on it. She was very discreet about this. No-one ever saw her take them, but she did, and she seemed to have great faith in them.

The doctors were delighted with her. She became a sort of "doctor's pet" for the senior AIDS doctor, a superb young woman, unbelievably dedicated to a task that was usually so unrewarding. Here was her pride and joy responding well to all these mysterious medications. She and Tarry loved and respected each other very much and continued to do so right to the end of Tarry's life.

A real thorn in Tarry's side, however, was her inability to work. She hated living on the invalid pension (in-valid pension she used to pronounce this), but she just didn't have the strength to commit herself to a job. Instead she turned to painting still life, scenery and portraits, some of which were very good indeed. The best of these was a portrait of her father, which would be presented to him on June 27, 1990, his 70th birthday. It had been painted from an old photograph, and was very moving. She made the frame herself, too. It hangs in pride of place in the front hall of our home in Kew, where it will always remain.

Tarry also had a wonderfully competent psychologist who really understood her needs and fears and hopes and dreams. Tarry felt very secure with this young woman. She suggested different kinds of activities for Tarry to pursue, mostly outdoors, but with the vagaries of Melbourne's weather kept in mind. So while things were good we went birdwatching, and Tarry climbed rocks high over Cape Schank, near Portsea, while, with my heart in my mouth, I looked on from below.

I only met this psychologist once or twice, but we were to have many, many long chats over the phone in the ensuing years, particularly when Caroline began to deteriorate. She was not a talker; she was a listener, a very good one – a God-given gift. When the chips are running out and time and life are slipping away from someone you love, the last thing you need is a garrulous ear-basher.

The rest of the family were settling down into their own lives again, and found they were comfortably able to answer any of their friends and acquaintances' questions about Caroline and AIDS. This made their friends more at ease with them, while at the same time these conversations were a means of dispelling some of the myths and falsehoods surrounding AIDS.

By now several months had passed since her first admission to hospital, and she had been back to hospital as both an outpatient and an inpatient. It was inevitable that the nature of her illness would become known.

The reactions of people were indeed quite interesting – varied to some degree, but with the common denominator of horror, grief and disbelief.

Some friends expressed their sorrow and support by very kindly sending flowers to us at home. I was very glad that Caroline was not here to see this happening. When the doorbell rang, I would answer it, and there would be yet another delivery of yet another bunch of flowers. It was making me very agitated because it seemed to me as though Caroline was dead already. I knew it was an expression of love and concern from those who, quite understandably, were unable to verbalize their feelings, but I just couldn't help wishing that those flowers were not arriving.

Other friends came around to our home and left casseroles with little notes on our doorstep. Again I felt it was almost as if Caroline had died. The food was very welcome, though, for I was spending so much time at Fairfield, in such a state of anxiety, that the household was in total disarray. I didn't have any outside help with the housework, let alone getting a meal on the table every night, so all contributions were indeed very gratefully accepted.

I felt extremely fortunate to have such practical and caring friends. Some were really very special. They were there, just right there, always around when I needed them. One friend used to drive me out to Fairfield when I felt I couldn't cope with the traffic back and forth each day. Another friend would ring up, not full of unsolicited advice, but just to chat and listen to me while I babbled on with lamentations of fear, sorrow, and a large measure of self pity. Yet other friends offered to have us stay with them on holiday interstate whenever we wished.

But, of course, there was a downside. Some folk stood back in horror and announced with dramatic flourishes that "There, but for the Grace of God, go I" and immediately disappeared from the scene, which was just as well, as I found that sort of reaction almost unbearable even though I know they didn't mean to be patronizing. The whole family certainly discovered who their real friends were at this time.

Frank's medical colleagues were also very supportive and genuinely sympathetic towards him. He was able to bury himself in his work for now. The time of retirement, a time that was to prove to be much more difficult for him, was still two years off. It was so hard for Frank, being a doctor. As a pathologist, he had spent many years looking down the microscope, diagnosing other people's diseases. His opinion was held in high regard, and his advice had been sought from time to time by overseas doctors who were having difficulties with some strange diagnoses, and very often Frank was able to come up with the right answers. But now, with his own daughter stricken with AIDS, there were no answers at all. There was nothing he could do, nothing he could find out. He was completely helpless. It was so sad and frustrating for him that all his years of study, thought and expertise were of no effect with HIV/AIDS.

I had, and still have, a very close friend from school days, living in America. In the ensuing years she was to send us many letters that contained cuttings from various newspapers, including the New York Times, Washington Post, and Guardian. These had the latest news of possible treatments and perhaps potential cures for AIDS, based on all kinds of experiments. We read them avidly and kept them in a special drawer in the hall table, hoping that one day some of these treatments would be available for Caroline. One or two of the drugs were eventually to be of some benefit to Caroline, but at a much later date.

A very distressing thing happened to me, and only to me, about two months after hearing the news of Caroline's illness. I got a series of really nasty anonymous phone calls. "Your Caroline has AIDS, has she? Ha Ha! Your time has come!" or words to that effect.

The caller was female and spoke only when I answered the phone. I did not recognize her voice, but we were to discover that she lived close by because in one phone call she said, "You went to Mass today, didn't you? But that won't cure Caroline." This was accompanied by laughter, then a click as the phone hung up.

We did eventually find out who this caller was, quite by chance. A middle-aged Catholic lady, she knew us, but not well. I did not confront her. I couldn't really, and I felt confrontation would only have added more stress to our lives, particularly mine. This unfortunate business said nothing for Catholic compassion, and it was very sad that this poor lady seemed to derive so much satisfaction from our misfortune.

By acquiring an unlisted phone number, we were able to ease that particular torment, although I still felt my comings and goings were under scrutiny. The seeds of future agoraphobic behavior in me had been sown.

After the change of phone number, things began to settle down once more. Going out to Fairfield became part of the daily routine. Caroline had adjusted to the naso-gastric feeding and was even putting on a little weight. She was still very apprehensive about what was happening to her, but enormously relieved that we were all rallying around her.

CHAPTER 4

⌇

A LEAKY BOAT

Things may have been going well for Caroline, but the family had now become worried about me. I wasn't aware of this at the time, at least not initially. They knew I was not coping, even though I could put on a reasonably good front when I had to. Socializing of any kind was becoming a nightmare; one glass of wine was enough to trigger an episode of crying. I was also smoking heavily and feeling rotten. I was still not able to see these warning signals, though. Apparently some of our friends were registering great alarm with the children and with Frank, but no-one said anything to me.

One source of stress was that it seemed as though all the decisions regarding Caroline were going to be left for me to deal with, phoning doctors about tests and adjustments in medications and similar things that I thought would have been better dealt with by Frank. He didn't want to worry the doctors, he said. He seemed to be distancing himself from the day to day realities of Caroline's illness and treatments and he was becoming rather remote towards me as well. It could have been his way of dealing with his own pain in those still early days of our association with AIDS. After all, it was only just over two months since our world had been shattered, then scattered all over the place, by this damned disease. My anxiety levels were increasing enormously, and still I did nothing about seeking help. I would come good eventually, I thought to myself.

Before I knew that Caroline was sick I had enrolled at LaTrobe University as a mature-aged student, to do a bachelor of arts degree. I had worked out that by working steadily it would take me about nine years to achieve this goal, by which time I would probably take out my degree in a wheelchair. For the first year I had chosen Italian language and European history, the topic of which was to be the French revolution. I had filled in the forms, been interviewed, and had passed the entrance exam. I was feeling very pleased with myself indeed. I had always liked to study and I really wanted to do a university course, and here was my big chance, at last.

It didn't work out at all, however. By the time the academic year had commenced in March 1989, Caroline was five months down the track with AIDS, and I was just as far down another track with anxiety. I simply couldn't manage all the assignments, reading, research and essays, although I forged on for two terms, dropping Italian along the way.

The lecturers and tutors were marvelous. They were so helpful and understanding. I had told them what had happened at home and they finally agreed that it was best if I discontinued the course. I did this, and felt some of the pressure lift from my shoulders, but a sense of failure was there as well.

Soon after leaving LaTrobe, I began showing very real signs of agoraphobia. It had been waiting to grab hold of me since the days of those sinister phone calls. I found myself unwilling, and then unable, to drive, even to the local shops, or to post a letter. I could not, literally could not, drive to the hairdresser in South Yarra. This hairdresser had become such a dear friend and confidant, as well as an expert in his trade, and he still is. He was well acquainted with AIDS, as many of his friends had died from it.

I feigned tiredness, or that Caroline was suddenly unwell, to avoid all outside activities, social or otherwise. I made a prison for myself behind the wrought iron front gates. I had to do this, I thought, in order to protect myself from the sight of other young people of Caroline's age who were all well and happy. They didn't have AIDS. Why didn't they have AIDS? Why was our Caroline the only girl we knew with AIDS? I was crying very often now, and I was frequently on my own at home. This was my fault, because I would not answer the front door for fear of anyone seeing that there really were chinks in the Joan Hurley armor.

It was at this point that Caroline stepped in and quite fearlessly, though tactfully, confronted me with the fact that I was in desperate need of medical help. I had helped her to a state of wellness, she said, and now she would help me to restore my life again. She had actually arranged everything, having collaborated with one of my most trusted and outspoken friends. They, or rather Caroline, had made an appointment for me to see a physician who was also a very close friend from St Vincents days. He had readily agreed to see me so, like a lamb to the slaughter, I meekly agreed to anything and everything.

Caroline herself drove me to Monash Medical Center, and having announced my arrival to the receptionist, quietly left for a coffee while I sat in the waiting room. It was full of anxious-looking young couples who apparently were unable to have babies and were possible candidates for the IVF (In Vitro Fertilization) program (the doctor I was to see is a very well-known and highly-regarded endocrinologist). I felt a bit out of place sitting there. I glanced at each couple and thought, I hope you are successful in your endeavors. I hope it will make you happy and, most of all, that you don't have troubles like our family does.

The doctor called me in, gave me a big comforting hug, told me I looked awful, but it was great to see me. He was still my friend after all these years! After examining me and talking to me for some time, he admitted that I was indeed in a great deal of trouble, physically and emotionally, which he thought was understandable under the circumstances. Much of this trouble was menopausal, a condition I hadn't given much thought to. The irregular periods and the mood swings had been around for some months, but I had not associated these with menopause, and did not realize that it could be treated. I did not know whether I had the "hot flushes" or not, because the feelings of fear and panic and anxiety left me constantly feeling hot one minute and cold the next.

A small dose of Hormone Replacement Therapy (HRT) was prescribed, and it was then very firmly suggested that I see a psychiatrist friend of the doctor. An appointment was made there and then for me to see this psychiatrist the next day at Royal Park.

Now I knew I really was in very big trouble. What else could be wrong with me? I was dizzy with shock and anxiety. Caroline drove me home. She was so gentle and kind to me. She took the HRT prescription up to the chemist, who delivered the tablets later that day, and I started on them right away. Caroline then set about organizing the evening meal.

The next day she drove me out to Royal Park Psychiatric Hospital. I was almost sick with apprehension. I knew virtually nothing about this branch of medicine except that if one was sick enough, one might be treated with electro-convulsive therapy (ECT). I had visions of Jack Nicholson's predicament in One Flew Over the Cuckoo's Nest.

Actually, the psychiatrist was wonderful to me, and after a hesitant beginning I was soon spilling out my tale of woe. I was telling him the most amazing things about myself; things hitherto long forgotten rose to the surface and popped out like bubbles in a fish tank. I was appalled and amazed. The doctor was not, even though I was painting what seemed to me the most awful verbal scenario.

After an hour and a half, which had flown by as quickly as a minute, my talking time was over. The doctor made various suggestions as to how to improve my lifestyle. For example, no alcohol, no cigarettes. I had to try to stop taking all the responsibility for Caroline's welfare. Although these very drastic immediate changes seemed a good idea, I didn't set too much store by them.

A course of some new anti-anxiety tablets was also prescribed for me. I was more than ready to try them out, something concrete and effective to help me at last. Caroline had the prescription made up very soon after driving me home from the hospital. I took the required dose three times daily for two days and nothing happened, nothing at all. I waited and waited through another day. Even after 72 hours, I was still as anxious as ever, so I had a glass of wine with the evening meal, took another tablet and felt even worse.

It turned out that this particular anti-anxiety agent takes a whole week to start its work of relieving symptoms. Well, of what use was that to me? I couldn't wait around one week for last Monday's anxiety to disappear on the following Monday. I stopped taking them altogether. I went back to the psychiatrist and he prescribed a small regular dose of a better known and widely used tablet, and this took effect almost immediately.

Throughout the first two weeks of treatment, in which I tried to get myself back on my feet, Caroline stayed right by my side, reassuring me, caring for me, comforting me with cups of tea and a shoulder to cry on. She did the shopping, washing, ironing and cooking. She did all of this with such care and affection. I felt really loved again. The roles had been reversed and Caroline was being my carer. How I loved her for loving me so much. And I knew then that eventually, perhaps soon, I would be really well, and therefore able to care for my darling girl for all her days in a rational and confident way. I could see and feel that I was gradually coming back to life again.

The following week, Frank suggested we all drive up to Queensland, to Surfers Paradise, for two weeks holiday. How fantastic! Caroline was really very well and happy and justifiably proud of what she had done for me. Frank was tired from work, as was Dominique, and Margie was free to join us also. Kristen was in Bali with her husband, and poor old Jamie was stuck with his "knives and forks" in the operating theater at Geelong Hospital.

We had to drive, as there had been a protracted pilots' strike which looked like going on forever. The trip wasn't too bad, but tempers were frayed from time to time during the long three-day haul from Melbourne. The main blessing was that Caroline stayed well, chirpy and very amusing.

In the first week Caroline, Margie and Dominique flew from Brisbane to Cairns and Cape Tribulation in an old Hercules aircraft. They had a wonderful time together and met up with some friends whom they had not seen for a very long time. None of these friends could believe that Caroline was ill, much less ill with AIDS. She was so full of excitement and adventure as they explored the rainforest and the beaches in perfect sunny weather. And all the while Caroline discreetly swallowed her tablets, on the dot of the appointed times every day. She kept the box of pills in an embroidered Mexican bag slung over her shoulder. Also in that bag was a thermometer just in case.

Frank and I, in the meantime, enjoyed our time alone together in the peace and quiet of sunshiny days and starlit nights. This helped to restore our rather ragged relationship. I think we had almost forgotten who we were.

The girls arrived back in Surfers Paradise looking brown, fit and sparkly-eyed and we all drove back home to Melbourne. We stopped over for one night in Corowa, the old home town of Frank's youth. His father had been the local doctor there for many years. He was able to show us the home in which he had been raised (when he wasn't boarding at Xavier College, Newman College and St Vincents Hospital). And many other places of deep nostalgia were also examined and admired.

It was to be the only time that Caroline would ever see the happy evidence of her beloved father's early days. This made it a very special and memorable trip. Thank God we took lots of photos.

A few days after our arrival home in Kew, another bomb was dropped on us, or more correctly, on Kristen. During their holiday in Bali, her husband had left her for a Balinese girl. Kristen had returned home alone. She and her husband had only been married just over 14 months.

The family was in total shock. We all closed ranks around Kristen to try to protect her from any further anguish on top of the terrible pain and grief and humiliation. Everyone seemed able to comfort her except me. I just couldn't do anything to help her. I looked at her and listened to her, and all the while I was thinking: "Oh no, you don't! I can't handle this, not another cross for me to bear. I can't help you carry this burden. Please don't ask me for help!" I wanted to run away.

Kristen is a very private person, not prone to emotional outbursts like her mother. She became very thin, pale, withdrawn and far too quiet. But all the while she handled the situation with grace, poise and such dignity, at enormous cost to her well-being. I will never cease to admire the fortitude and courage she showed during that time of tragedy in her life. She kept her pain and sorrow mostly to herself.

A wonderfully kind and very competent solicitor took over, and thanks to him, the divorce was resolved as quickly and painlessly as possible. Kristen reverted to her maiden name, bought a dear little house of her own, and started a new life along with a menagerie of dogs and cats and a very pleasant lodger.

She achieved this all on her own. Perhaps it was for the best that I was hardly involved at all during that time, for it showed that Kristen's independence was intact. But even to admit that made me realize once and for all that I simply had to do something drastic to pull myself together totally. I had to bring myself closer to each of my children and not just to Caroline. The others had hardly received more than a passing thought during the previous year. Certainly the doctors and their medications had helped me, but I had to do something by myself to complete my healing. I puzzled over what I could do.

The ability to pray formally, apart from spontaneous supplications such as "Oh God, don't let Caroline die, please make her well again," had long since left me. I hated going to Mass, especially after one priest, lips pursed and face puckered with distaste, had announced during his homily that we must have compassion for "our poor brothers struck down by that killer disease AIDS." No mention of sisters, I noted. Mentally I yelled at him, "Shut up! You patronizing old preacher man." I got up and walked out of the church, trembling with indignation. And I didn't go back, except for weddings, of course.

One Saturday morning late in September I was having a cup of tea and reading the supplement to one of the Melbourne newspapers when an advertisement caught my eye. It was for a course in relaxation and therapeutic massage that was to be held part-time for one year at a well-known and highly-regarded school of massage located in Camberwell, just five minutes from Kew.

That was it. This, I realized, was exactly what I had been looking for. Forget the academic aspirations and do something I knew I was capable of doing. This course would be interesting, time-consuming and physically demanding, just perfect for me. Without realizing it, I had unlocked the gates that released me from agoraphobia for good.

Having made an appointment for an interview with the director, I drove over to the school, and to my delight, I was accepted. I think the nursing background helped. The classes were to be held every Thursday afternoon and on one weekend each month. There would be many written and practical assignments, with examinations at the end of the year. It was all to be taken very seriously and professionally in order to stamp out the stigma attached to massage because of its sexual connotations.

I bought all the books and equipment and could hardly wait to start the course in March 1990. This was such a positive thing to do, I reasoned. It was something that would be of great benefit to me and as I acquired the skills of massage, I would be able to benefit others, especially sick others, a prediction that would later turn out to be true.

It seemed no time at all before Christmas was coming around again, and it was such a joy with Tarry so well. We had just given Kristen a really great 30th birthday party, with lots of her friends and much fun and good cheer. I felt a bit sheepish about the lack of concern I had shown her, but being the innately good and kind girl that she is, Kristen seemed to have forgiven me.

My sister made the Christmas puddings this time. Tarry and I drove out to a Christmas tree farm where we selected a nicely shaped tree that was chopped down and secured in the boot of the car for the drive home. It was our first real Christmas tree in years.

While Tarry and I drove slowly along Warrigal Road towards Kew, the tree started to dislodge itself from the boot. The ropes had slipped. I couldn't stop laughing as Tarry tried to direct me into a side street in order to secure the tree back into position. It was hilarious, and once again, it was Tarry who fixed it up and completed the drive home.

We placed the tree upright, holding it securely with bricks in a bucket of water, which we then covered in tin foil as a decorative touch. Next we invited all the family, my sister and her girls and a few close friends, to help decorate this wondrous tree with myriad baubles, trinkets and lights. Tarry had made a large and beautifully colored lead-light star, which was suspended by a length of fishing line from the ceiling directly over the top of the tree. Tarry's star was never taken down and will remain there to hover over all future Christmas trees. We had a little champagne party around the tree to celebrate this momentous occasion.

Christmas Day was a total triumph. All the family were gathered together once again, including a few young people who had no families of their own with whom to celebrate. Tarry, I have to say, was the Christmas star personified that year. She bustled around, clearing the table, bringing in the pudding all lit up with sparklers. She chortled away with all the folks, ate everything in sight, and happily enter-tained the next-door neighbor's children when they called in after lunch with their own little ones. Oh, what a truly blessed day that was.

A week later, on New Year's Eve, it was Dominique's birthday. I felt this was the time to make her feel really special by giving her a rollicking Hurley-style party. Dominique had had an awful year. She was unhappy with the catering course she was doing. She was very upset about Tarry having AIDS, and her personal life had been unhappily erratic. She had endured it all with hardly a passing word of comfort from her miserable old mum. Perhaps she would think this party a peace offering.

In a way I suppose it was. But Dominique didn't seem to mind; she is a very understanding girl and she and I have always been great friends. I loved her so much for being so patient with me. Anyway, it was a fabulously successful birthday party regardless of the party giver's motive!

Tarry celebrated her 29th birthday with her friends at a Thai restaurant in Brunswick. At her request, she organized it, but she seemed uncomfortable at being the center of attention. I really think she would have enjoyed it more had Frank and I not been there. Our presence cramped her rather hippie style somewhat, especially as she was still so well and certainly didn't need to be watched over.

The summer rolled happily by at Portsea, during which time I made a final and momentous decision regarding myself. On February 26, 1990, I gave up cigarettes and alcohol forever. It was the best decision I have ever made for me and for those close to me. "Annus Horribilis" 1989 was over for me forever (with apologies for stealing a line from Her Majesty Queen Elizabeth II). I have never looked back since that day, and I have never missed either the wine or the cigarettes, not even for a minute.

Within two weeks I felt fantastic, and started to look well, too. My eyes were clear and bright again, and the anxiety just fell away. My body lost its puffy look and became trim once more. I think drinking lots of mineral water (1.5 liters of Evian) each day helped with this remarkable transformation. I couldn't believe it and it took all the family and friends by surprise. Their flattering remarks made me feel wonderful. Their relief was great, particularly that of Frank and Tarry, who had done most of the worrying, I'm sorry to say.

My life swung into a new and hopeful curve upwards. I knew now that I would definitely be able to cope with just about anything that came along, which was just as well, for when things did go wrong, they would do so quickly and dramatically, but I knew what to do, and more importantly, what not to do.

Chapter 5

Steady as She Goes

As 1990 swung into gear, Tarry's vigor remained constant. Her weight was almost normal and her T-cells were at an adequately high level. (Personally I am against AIDS patients knowing their T-cell count, for once the T-cell count drops, never to rise again, quite often these patients give up the fight and abandon hope of ever being or feeling well again.)

Tarry was also very convinced of the benefits of alternative therapies. Eastern medicine, herbs and massage were equally as important to her as western medication and she stuck religiously with both forms of healing. She loved the massages I had learned to give her and she also felt the benefit of Chinese acupuncture, carried out by a totally AIDS-aware and unprejudiced Chinese doctor in Fitzroy, a wonderful man.

Tarry had a deep and abiding faith in eastern philosophy and spirituality. She read many books covering these topics and attended lectures, many given by a friendly and understanding group of Tibetan monks. Buddhism provided her favored form of spiritual comfort. And she managed quite skillfully to maintain a balanced approach to both eastern and western religions and medicines. This was to be of great solace to her right up to the time she died.

Yoga and meditation were also high on Tarry's agenda for keeping well, and each day she devoted at least one hour to these practices. There was a stillness and peace surrounding her which created an atmosphere of ease and harmony among those she mingled with from day to day. Her family, friends and even fellow patients and medical staff all noticed this aura around Tarry. It was almost tangible at times.

Where once Tarry had been a total vegetarian, now everything that was of nutritional value was included in her diet. Jamie's future wife,

Sally, was a capable dietitian who helped us sort out what was good and suitable for maintaining Tarry's weight. Chinese herbs also featured on the menu. What hideous things Tarry would boil up in my biggest saucepan: herbs, roots and strange things that looked like "eye of newt" and "wing of bat" or whatever the witches in Macbeth brewed up in their cauldron of spells. They would have been most impressed with Tarry's efforts. After simmering this lot for some time, the whole revolting mess was strained, cooled and Tarry would drink it.

By now March had come and gone and I was well into the massage course. It was all that I had hoped for and more. My fellow students were mostly quite young and we all got along famously together. It was especially good for me to be anonymous. No-one knew anything about me or I them. I could relax, be myself and have fun, as well as learn the wonderful, healing, soothing massage techniques. I was in heaven.

There was one, and only one, reference to AIDS in all of that wonderful year. It was a question about whether it was safe to massage a client who had HIV or AIDS. My heart stood still. The answer came back to this effect: it was perfectly safe as long as there were no open cuts on either masseur or client. And anyway, how was one to know who had HIV or not among everyday clients who appeared to be in good health? And that was the end of that.

My fellow students and I were like a bunch of school children in our enthusiastic effort to have an A+ marked in red ballpoint on our written assignments, and at least a credit for the examinations. I think I completed the year knowing more about surface anatomy and the human skeleton than my doctor husband and son.

More good things were happening within the family, all of whom were well, happy, relaxed and getting on with life's daily business. Margie was leaving for America in May, to do her Master of Law degree at the George Washington University in Washington DC. Her major was to be environmental law, and she would be away for one year. This was all courtesy of the law firm for whom Margie worked as a solicitor.

It was such an honor and we were all so pleased for her, especially Tarry, with whom Margie had a special rapport. They had traveled extensively together prior to the onset of AIDS. I knew Tarry was apprehensive about Margie being away for so long but she hid this fear quite well.

Margie had a marvelous new man in her life, the man she would eventually marry and whom we all loved. A gentle, kind man, he adored his Margie and showed great affection toward us all, especially his friend and cohort, Tarry. Peter would travel to the USA with Margie to get her organized and settled into the course as well as do some legal work there. So yet another party was held to farewell the two of them. We seemed to be always celebrating something, and we loved it. I used to enjoy entertaining before the troubles, so it was wonderful to feel really well again and able to continue this Hurley tradition of celebrating everything in sight.

Tarry was home at Kew only rarely these days. Her state of health was very good, so she spent most of her time at Brunswick. She kept her regular outpatients appointments for checkups at Fairfield by herself. At these times her medication status was reviewed and supplies were replenished. Huge paper bags filled with bottles and blister packs, even jars of pills, were all carried home for sorting out.

Winter was now approaching, and Tarry grew quite anxious and afraid. She really was terrified of the cold, and I was fearful for her. After Tarry died, I discovered among her things a letter to a friend in France, in which she had written that the dank and darkness of a Melbourne winter was the ideal environment for disease to grow and fester. She longed to live in the sun. For although Tarry appreciated having the use of our beach house at Portsea to escape from Melbourne, whatever the season, it was the warmth of the sun that she craved.

In that early winter of 1990, I remember Tarry planting daffodil and jonquil bulbs under the big, old golden poplar tree in the center of our front lawn. While she was doing this, she wondered out loud to me if she would live to see them flower the following spring. She did live to see the fruits of her labor, and would for the next three springs. Each year, as they self-propagate, more and more daffodils and jonquils appear, spreading over the lawn, a living memorial quilt of gold and yellow which returns to us each year as a reminder of our beloved Tarry's presence among us still.

Tarry loved the quotation from The Rubaiyat of Omar Khayyam which said: *Come fill the cup and in the fire of spring, the winter garment of repentance fling.*

Before the real chill of winter set in we went on a shopping spree to buy thermal underwear and lots of winter garments for Tarry: jumpers, leggings, tights, skivvies, socks, scarves, pants, woolen hats and a brand new fleecy-lined parka. She looked and felt marvelous. We brought home all the carry bags to gloat over their contents. Frank pretended to have a heart attack when he surveyed the damage we had done with the credit card. Such are the joys of retail therapy.

Tarry also had the anti-flu injection to help ward off any sinister and life-threatening AIDS-related conditions that were lurking around. There were many deaths among the men with AIDS that winter. We still did not know of any other women with the same condition. Luckily for Tarry she was spared any illness at all during that winter. She kept busy with her painting, gardening and reading, and seeing her many friends.

About this time in 1990 all the family were enjoying a certain amount of stability in their lives, although each of us was very aware of the real situation. It was now over 12 months since Tarry had been in hospital, and she actually seemed to be making some progress. Well, she wasn't regressing in any apparent way. The doctors considered her to be their 'star' patient. She was cooperative and dependable and had enormous family backup.

With my troubles well behind me, I was really enjoying my massage course. Kristen was very happy and settled in her career as a medical scientist in hematology and was planning a trip to America to see Margie, who was happily engrossed in her post graduate studies. Jamie had successfully completed his first examination for the Fellowship of the Australian College of Surgeons. Everything in the garden seemed quite rosy.

Frank and I were so buoyed up by this that we began to plan a six week holiday overseas in March 1991. It was so exciting. The main drawcard was the prospect of visiting Margie in her flat in Washington DC. We both missed her terribly, although she was remarkably good at keeping in touch by way of frequent and lengthy reverse-charge phone calls.

We also wanted to visit San Francisco General Hospital, where there was an enormous department devoted to AIDS. We hoped we could get more information regarding the availability of drugs and treatment that might be useful for Caroline. We were also very interested to see if American AIDS care was more up to date than that in Australia. We were to discover that there certainly was a greater level of AIDS awareness in the States, but we really were not in a position to judge which country provided the better care.

We had obtained Caroline's AIDS history or Curriculum Vitae from Fairfield. Under "Cause of Illness" were the letters IVDU. I didn't know what that meant. I asked Jamie and he told me it was Intravenous Drug Use, so yet another shock, and a few more pieces of the puzzle fell into place. It became apparent to me then that Caroline's adventurous travels, which had drawn her to remote areas of the world, had included another more treacherous path that would lead her to her untimely death. She had unwittingly chosen the wrong path, from which there were no safe refuges. Her perilous journey along the road began in Morocco, Portugal and Spain in 1982-83. A decade later she would be dead. Not that any of us had a clue about that at that time.

I didn't confront her with my newly-acquired knowledge, of course, but much later she would tell me all about her life and the travels which had included these dangerous activities.

CHAPTER 6

༈

SUBMERGED REEF AHEAD

By early September, 1990, winter was almost over and Tarry had come through unharmed. Things changed dramatically and suddenly on Tuesday, September 11, when she arrived home at Kew with a raging temperature, chest pains and a hacking cough. She had driven herself from Brunswick and was in a terrible state. I rang Fairfield, and she was admitted immediately into Ward Five. I was very frightened for her, but this time there was no panic. Just as well, for Tarry had contracted the hitherto dreaded pneumocystic carinii pneumonia (PCP), which had taken the lives of many young men with AIDS in recent times.

Tarry seemed to be more disappointed than frightened by this new and sudden turn of events. She appeared not to be harboring any thoughts of death this time, and she responded well and quickly to massive doses of antibiotics. Her difficulty with swallowing returned, so she was back onto the naso-gastric tube feeding for some time.

This illness was to mark her return yet again to the treadmill of a few days in hospital, home, then hospital again. During one of her respite stays at Kew another angry rash appeared all over her body. Fortunately, it was not nearly as bad as the first episode in October 1988. She had built up quite a tolerance to Bactrim. But even so, the dosage had to be reduced to clear up the rash. More gradually the PCP cleared up too, thank God.

A contributory factor to Tarry's PCP episode, it turned out, was that for some weeks Tarry had ceased taking AZT, having volunteered to go onto the trial drug DDI. Her system had to be cleared of other anti-AIDS agents before commencing DDI, which was being studied at the Brompton Hospital in London, and was being sent from the UK to Australia. Unfortunately this drug had not arrived in Australia at the appropriate time for Tarry to start taking it and too much time had elapsed following the cessation of AZT. I was seething with rage when I found out. I tore strips off one of the attending doctors. And she, only young and new at Fairfield, was just as furious with me.

"Caroline will die and it will be your fault," I yelled at her at the entrance to the ward. The poor young doctor just walked away.

This episode caused quite a commotion, which both amused and embarrassed Tarry. One of Jamie's friends, a doctor in the research department, pacified me and reassured me that Tarry would be alright. The Anglican pastoral care sister came to the rescue, as she had so kindly done so many times, and would again in the coming years. I later apologized profusely, but the doctor avoided me altogether after that.

The DDI arrived on Monday, October 8, 1990. Tarry very bravely swallowed her first dose. It was a revolting gelatinous powder that came in a sachet with "for clinical trials only" stamped on it. It was mixed with a glass of water and had to be taken immediately. I think Tarry was the only female taking this drug. Once again we were on the lookout for side effects.

Her skin color deepened to resemble a rather orange-tinted suntan. It was not altogether unattractive, but she was to become tired of remarks alluding to the fact that she had had too much sun and might get skin cancer. A minimal hair loss was apparent, but that didn't worry Tarry. She was pinning her hopes on the DDI, which was later available in tablet form, making it much more palatable and easy to take. She was still taking her "witches brew" along with all her other medications, most of which she had been taking for exactly two years now.

By mid-October we were beginning to think that the DDI was going to prove a breakthrough. Tarry seemed to be remarkably well, and even suggested that I have a small lunch party for a few of my supportive friends, some of whom had very serious family problems of their own. Tarry helped – and she was fantastic. Everyone cast aside their worries for a few precious hours. It was an unqualified success and I am so glad I had that gathering then, especially with Tarry there. But I could not muster up the strength to repeat the performance, for most of the next two years were to be horrific for Caroline and for us all.

Some weeks later Tarry again began to feel extremely unwell. She was admitted to Fairfield for investigations into her recurrent high fever, sore throat and chest, and stomach pain. A gastroscopy was performed on her. These mild symptoms of various complaints came and went. But one complaint never went away, and was the cause of much distress for Tarry. This condition was called mycobacterial avium complex or "MAC," as it is known in the AIDS community. It is a type of tubercular infection allied to true tuberculosis but less sensitive to normal anti-tubercular drugs. Tarry would have contracted this as a residual infection from the early days of the AIDS-related tuberculosis diagnosed in October 1988. There was no specific treatment available for this ailment at that time, so Tarry had no alternative but to continue taking her original anti-tubercular medication.

Tarry, with her indomitable spirit, accepted this as part of the rotten old AIDS package and got on with life as best she could. She kept as active as possible, swimming, cycling and walking, and she was an avid reader. The Lord of the Rings was her favorite. But she needed to rest a lot, and sometimes almost entire days were spent sleeping. These days really worried me, because I had always understood that people with serious illnesses who slept a great deal during the day were drawing very close to death. But there again, there was no telling with the AIDS virus. It teases and torments both the patient and the carer, like a cheeky little demon bringing terror one day and hope the next. You really never know what to expect, so it is of paramount importance to maintain a balance between being calm and relaxed, and at the same time remaining on full alert. This is a skill you make yourself acquire as you move from one situation to the next. One really can do anything if one has to.

The week before Tarry started on the DDI drug trial, Dominique had flown off to Spain to do a three month course learning Spanish at the University of Salamanca. It seemed to me a long way to go to have a dabble in acquiring new language skills but she was almost panicky in her insistence on getting away from home. She had enough money, she said, and she had certainly had a bad year, so off she went on September 25, 1990. As she had been to Spain before, I wasn't really worried about her, particularly as she was to be billeted with a family near the university and would be home some time after Christmas.

What did worry me was the fact that I was losing another member of my closest support group. Three months may not seem long, but with AIDS, time has no meaning. The virus can rear up into a fatal illness in three days or lie dormant for another three years. There was no telling what might happen. With Dominique gone and Margie in America, I was really on my mettle to remain calm and in control while I watched Tarry closely for adverse reactions to this unknown DDI drug. Kristen and Jamie were always supportive. Even so, they were tied up with long working hours at their respective jobs. Of course, Kristen was still to heal completely from her broken marriage, broken heart and divorce.

Christmas was rapidly approaching. This year Tarry was not well enough to come with me to the Christmas tree farm. As it seemed a worthy alternative to support a good cause, we purchased a tree from Community Aid Abroad, which was delivered to our home. We have done the same each Christmas since. My sister and her family came for Christmas lunch, which certainly helped fill the gaps created by the absence of Margie and Dominique. It was a happy and comfortable day, and provided an excellent opportunity to farewell Kristen in style. She was flying off to America on Boxing Day for four weeks, a well-earned holiday. She was traveling with a close friend and was really looking forward to seeing Margie in Washington DC in addition to experiencing some of the attractions that America has to offer.

Three of the five children would now be out of the country and Tarry, although happy for them, was quite understandably very jealous. She was furious that she would never be well enough to travel again. I felt so sad for her, for she had always loved her journeys around the world. She had packed a lot of traveling into a short space of time, though, and when the opportunity arose, and if she was well enough, there was still plenty to do and see in Australia. This, too, would prove to present problems, for when later she did travel far from Melbourne and became ill, the appropriate help was quite often not available, and on one occasion was actually withheld because Tarry had AIDS. On that occasion, I stepped in and demanded, shrieked and carried on until she was given what she needed. It was very upsetting.

After Christmas, Frank and I went to Portsea, suggesting to Tarry that she visit whenever she felt like driving down. We didn't want her to feel trapped by insisting that she come with us. The weather was superb, very warm and beachy, so Tarry was with us more often than not. She really enjoyed the long, lazy days on her beloved Portsea back beach and at London Bridge.

I had successfully completed the massage course in December 1990, and was planning to set up my own practice, working from home in Kew after our trip. While at Portsea, I was offered the opportunity to stand in for a very good local masseuse who practiced there full-time all year round and was anxious to have a 10 day holiday herself. I agreed to do this, albeit rather nervously at first.

I became more confident each day and I loved the job. It was a wonderful experience. The clients were all friendly and most appreciative and those on holidays later came to me in Melbourne. I was indeed fortunate to have been given such a marvelous opportunity to test the waters of what would hopefully be a new career. And I loved earning some money of my own, which I secreted away to spend on our trip.

During her visits to Portsea I always gave Tarry a massage, and after having spent a day in the surf and sun, she would love this. I was very happy to observe that she was still quite well covered, no apparent weight loss or changes in her skin. This happy state of affairs lasted throughout that summer.

Frank and I now felt safe to finalize our plans for our trip to America and England. Passports were renewed, visas obtained and airline bookings made. First class, no less. I was so excited. Although having traveled abroad a few times before, I had never done so in such style. "First class is madness," Frank had said. But I didn't agree. "You can't take it with you," I replied. It was later pointed out to me that I had made quite sure we couldn't. I was a very reliable spendthrift on that wonderful holiday.

Dominique had arrived home on January 7. Much to our delight, she looked very well and was all glowing and happy again. She seemed to have found renewed purpose in her life. Tarry was particularly pleased to see her, as she was very anxious to have first-hand news of her beloved Spain. They spoke Spanish together quite frequently for a while, but with time, most of the linguistic gymnastics faded away.

By the end of January Tarry's health was really much improved. She looked very well too. The ailments that had been niggling at her insides

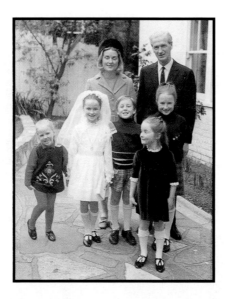

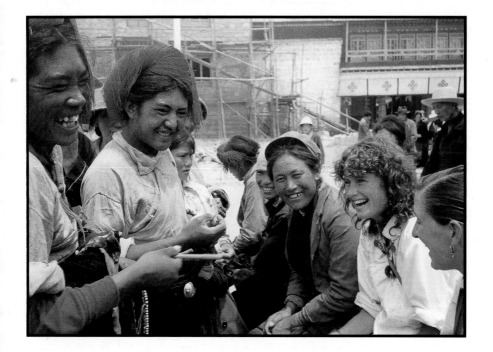

ABOVE: *Caroline's First Communion Day*
         left to right: Dominique, Caroline, Jamie, Margie and Kristen, back: Joan and Frank
BELOW: *Caroline (second from right) with her friends in Tibet, 1986*

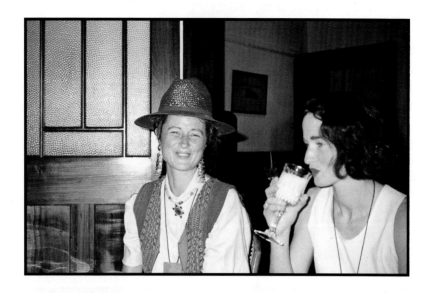

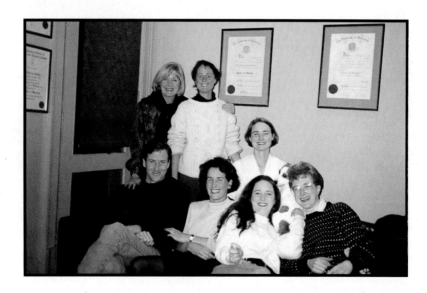

ABOVE: *Caroline in South American clothes, hamming it up with Margie,*
        Christmas morning at Kew, 1990
BELOW: *Family gathering 1991 - Jamie and Sally are engaged*
        back: Joan and Caroline, middle: Margie
        front: Jamie, Sally, Dominique and Kristen

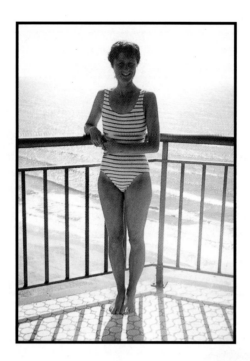

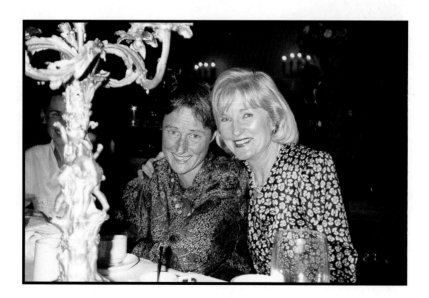

ABOVE: *Caroline at Surfers Paradise, 1990*
BELOW: *Caroline and Joan at Mietta's Restaurant, 1991*

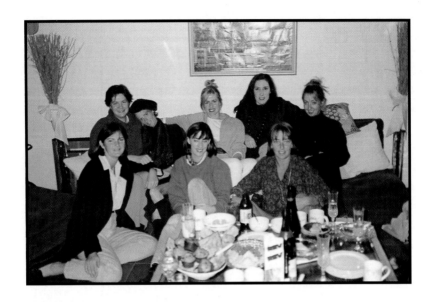

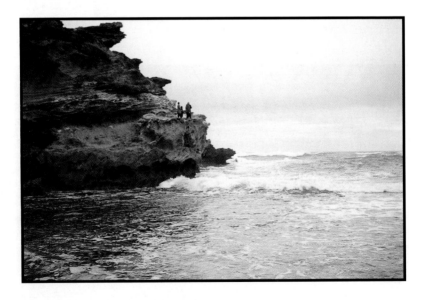

ABOVE: *Caroline, now weak and thin, with her beloved "Card Girls", May 16th 1993*
        back row: Anna, Caroline, Helen, Frances, Sally
        front row: Kate, Sarah and Kerrie
BELOW: *Family scattering Caroline's ashes into the ocean from London Bridge,*
        Portsea, Victoria, July 4th 1993

seemed to have settled down. She was happier in herself and clearly seemed pleased that Frank and I were going away for a seven-week holiday. We had not left her since her illness was diagnosed, but she and I knew she would be safe with so many caring family members, relatives and friends who knew exactly what to do if anything should go wrong. It also boosted her feeling of independence, and made her feel that she really couldn't be too ill if we were confident about leaving her so far behind. I must admit I felt considerably more wobbly about this than I appeared. But we owed it to ourselves to take this holiday and we were only a plane flight away, after all.

Another reason for feeling free and confident enough to plan a trip abroad was the knowledge that Caroline would be safe within the security of the unique and wonderful family of Fairfield Hospital. It was ready at all times, day and night, to enfold her in the familiar arms of the medical care so trusted by Caroline. She would not be swallowed up in a huge institution, of which the section devoted to AIDS might be quite small.

Fairfield was a homey hospital; loving, warm, and unique. The specially trained nurses, and all the associated staff, from doctors to domestics (not necessarily in that order), were all there to take care of these special, fragile, patients. This was the one and only hospital where fear of the environment was out of place and virtually unknown. Had this not been the case, we would never have left Caroline's side, not even for one minute, because the chances of another ARC attacking were very real and ever present. Thus the safe haven of Fairfield was very reassuring for Caroline, for us, and for her sisters and brother who would be watching over her during our absence.

Kristen arrived home at the end of January looking refreshed, relaxed and happy. So all was very well indeed.

The date of our departure was March 9, 1991. I had the suitcases, one each, packed and ready to go on Saturday, February 23. I was as organized and eager as Tarry used to be for her travels. There was one difference, though. My case was packed with conventional clothing for all occasions. Tarry's backpack, on the other hand, would have been sparsely packed with sturdy, casual clothing, one good skirt and top thrown in just in case.

We had chosen early March as the time to go because Frank was due to retire on Friday, March 1. Although he had known for five years that this was going to happen, I don't think he ever really believed that the dreaded day would come. When it did, it was accompanied by a terrible sense of shock and sadness, a type of grief at having to leave behind his beloved microscope and all those years of happy service to medicine. To make things even worse, Frank would now be at home all day, every day, and this would mean being continually exposed to the gradual deterioration of his beloved Tarry, a cross that would be almost too heavy a burden for him to bear.

The timing of the trip was therefore important. We would set off exactly one week after his wonderful, but sad farewell dinner, held for him by his colleagues at the Melbourne Club.

On the day of our departure, we said our rather tearful goodbyes at Kew. I didn't want any emotional scenes at Tullamarine airport. After all the usual ticketing, passport and customs routines were completed, we were called onto the plane. We settled ourselves into the large and comfortable first class seats and stretched out our legs (such acres of space around us, I couldn't believe it). As we accepted the slim crystal flute of Laurent-Perrier champagne, Frank and I looked at each other, smiled and held hands. I knew I still really loved him, in spite of all the tension there had been between us since October 13, 1988. I have always remembered that special moment, because the tension was to become much worse as Tarry drew closer to death; we would be virtually no help to each other at all during the last few weeks of her life.

The door of the aircraft closed, sealing us off from the fears and traumas of home. We were on our way at last. I placed a pillow behind my head, reclined the seat and released the seatbelt. I was ready to indulge in the delicious anticipation of the places and people we would be seeing which were to bring us so much joy in the coming seven weeks. But Tarry crept into my mind; her travels had been so important to her and the memories of those times came flooding back to me.

Just as the plane to America from Australia took us back in time when we crossed the date line, so my mind returned to Caroline's traveling days and to the time before the journey through AIDS began.

CHAPTER 7

∽

DISTANT SHORES

Tarry's taste for travel had come about as a result of a cruel blow to her aspirations for a career in graphic arts. Her last year at school was 1978, when she completed her Higher School Certificate with adequate marks to undertake a graphic arts course. She had no academic ambitions and was an average student, but she had a creative and imaginative side to her character; she really loved art and was good at it. She was delighted to be accepted into an introductory year in graphic arts at a technical college in Prahran.

Tarry's natural enthusiasm swung into top gear. She loved the challenge of the course and the opportunities it gave her to demonstrate in her folio her ability to design with harmony, color and coordination, and originality. She received commendation for her work during her next year, 1980, at another technical college in Hawthorn, and was very happy indeed with the prospect of completing the course there.

Then quite out of the blue, her course had come to an abrupt halt when the head of the graphic arts department told her that she would not be accepted to do her final year. It had generally been considered that her folio was not up to the required standard. This came as a terrible and totally unexpected shock to Tarry and to all of us too.

Not a single hint had been given to her, and she was informed that "no further correspondence would be entered into." Efforts by her father to determine exactly what was going on failed to elicit any answers. With one strike of a bureaucrat's pen, Tarry was cut off from the course she really loved, a course to which she had devoted so much time and effort, and which she had been so close to completing. She had been confident, and up until then had been told she was good at her work – but not quite good enough, it seemed.

Tarry's self-esteem took a terrible dive. She could not understand why this had happened to her when everything seemed to be progressing so well. We talked about it for hours on end, but no amount of encouraging words would console her. She wept and wept while we all racked our brains trying to think of an acceptable alternative – acceptable to Tarry, that is. She needed something to help her up and over her very real sense of failure.

Looking back to the end of 1980 and to this never adequately explained rejection of her strenuous and enthusiastic efforts in a field for which she appeared to have a natural aptitude, I firmly believe that this episode represents a turning point in Tarry's life. It destroyed something of her previous trust in people, because throughout the year she spent at this institution she had experienced nothing but encouragement and fairly regular commendation for her efforts. It was an enormous blow to her confidence.

Tarry knew, and Frank and I knew, that she did not have the intellectual ability of her sisters or brother. This never worried her in the slightest. The elevated streams of university and academic life held no attractions for her. She just loved art and things artistic with a passion. This rejection (and Tarry was well aware that many others had suffered the same fate) was not one that hurt her pride, but it left a cruel dent in her faith in those she did not know well. Her reaction was simply to abandon study and to embrace experience.

After a period of righteous rage and anger, Tarry set her sights on traveling, not following the usual tourist tracks, but taking those that led her to more mysterious and less well-known countries. A small fire had been lit in her, and eventually it would fan into a bonfire of desire for adventurous travel.

The money to do this was earned by working with a catering firm from dawn to dusk and beyond, as kitchen hand, then sandwich-maker, moving gradually up to silver service waitressing. She was her jolly old self again by this time, and absolutely hell bent on earning every cent she could. She seemed happy in the service too, and looked the part in her white shirt and long black skirt.

Tarry used to practice the difficult and cumbersome silver-service style of waitressing here at home, with me posing as the guests.

She would set 10 places at our round breakfast-room table, with a dinner plate in each setting. Tarry would then load up a large silver tray with, for example, mushrooms, carrots, peas, potatoes and chicken pieces, all in separate mounds on the tray. Then with white-gloved right hand she would quite skillfully manage a silver spoon and fork while her left hand and arm supported the tray.

She would serve my dinner 10 times as I moved from one seat to the next. It was very arduous for her, but good practice and great for a laugh (at home, not at work) and I only ever had one or two mushrooms or baby carrots tipped down the front of my shirt. Luckily the real dinner guests were not subjected to the same fate.

Within 12 months, by scrimping and saving, and with more than a little help from her father, Tarry had enough money to finance her first trip to South America. Her friends, three girls of her own age, which at that time was 19, had flown off a week before. Tarry was to meet them in Mexico City.

She accomplished this with no difficulty at all, for she was very well prepared, both psychologically and physically. She had done extensive reading about the various South American countries she was to visit, and thus had a good idea of what to expect, and she was very fit as well. Tarry was quite a fitness fanatic – always exercising, swimming, bike riding and bush walking, to name but some of the activities she indulged in.

Frank and I had arranged a pre-travel meeting at home with the parents of Tarry's traveling companions to make sure that everyone knew what they were doing and when and where they were going. We were all relieved to find that each member of the group had at least one person or family member they could contact in each South American country on their itinerary.

It was still with a great deal of apprehension, however, that we waved Tarry off at Tullamarine on December 14, 1980. When the passport control doors closed firmly behind her, I had these twinges of fear that I was losing the Tarry I had always known, and that a different, altered Caroline would return to us in two months time.

After meeting up with her friends, Tarry rang us reverse charges from Mexico City. She thanked us very warmly for helping her to get launched and sounded quite dithery with excitement. The eight-week adventure stretched out before her, and she was ready to go and enjoy it and taste real and glorious freedom for the first time. She could, and would, see and do everything possible.

It was this first trip that was to sow the seeds of her insatiable desire to seek out and savor the little-known and ancient mysteries of foreign lands, a desire that would bring about changes in Tarry that would remain with her permanently. Never again would she settle down and live at home for any length of time. There was too much to see and do elsewhere. While she would always be loving and caring towards her family and friends, the call for new adventures would keep bearing her away.

She was an intrepid traveler and fear never seemed to deter her. Having followed a route from Mexico to Belize, through Guatemala and Nicaragua to Colombia, she then ventured on to Ecuador and Peru. She was completely overwhelmed by the Andes and deeply fascinated by the Aztecs. Her one regret was not getting to Chile.

During the trip, Tarry kept a very detailed and beautifully written diary. She entered into this exercise book each day's experiences of the scenic splendors she saw, the people she met, and the food, culture, art, architecture and politics of each place she visited. It also detailed her delight in trying out marijuana, which was readily available from the locals. Her delicious freedom gave her the scope to do as she pleased and it was her decision to try anything, albeit infrequently.

In the case of marijuana, even though she found it relaxing and a fun thing to do with friends, it was too expensive to indulge in too often, it seems. She also wrote in her diary that she disliked wasting her time recovering from the effects. Because I did not have access to this diary until many years later, I had absolutely no clue as to what was going on.

I was delighted simply that she was thoughtful enough to ring whenever she could, which was not often, and that she was having such a good time. Those calls were eagerly awaited by us and were the cause of enormous joy when we heard her cheery voice competing with the crackly connections from some remote area. She always sounded so happy, and although she often thought of us all, she was not in any hurry to catch the return flight on February 8, 1981.

On her return, and for years following, Tarry wrote colorful letters to a French friend and fellow traveler, Anouck, who sent me copies after Tarry died.

March 1981

Dear Anouck,

It was fantastic to hear from you. Your letter brought all the memories back which are fading fast. I got back to Australia on the 8th February, and already Mexico seems like years ago...

Wasn't Belize amazing? We really loved it. Don't you agree it was a great change from Mexico? Peta and I spent three days there, then left and went to Tikal.

Tikal was just beautiful. It was great sleeping outdoors in hammocks, surrounded by that incredible jungle. We went as far as Sobla from Lake Arittan.

We flew from Guatemala to Bogota arriving there at midnight, which was very scary. On the plane we were told to remove all jewelry because it could be ripped from us by the locals.

We were also warned against catching taxis as the drivers couldn't be trusted. What made things worse was that we had no local money and all the exchange bureaus at the airport were closed! In the end we decided to sleep at the airport for the night.

Next morning we met a Columbian whose wife and two children had just left for Australia. He drove us to friends of Mum and Dads who live in Bogota. We spent a week with them in their tiny little farm house half an hours drive from the city up in the mountains.

We had a wonderful time with them and saw, as well as experienced the life-style of a Columbian family.

It was very sad to say goodbye to them as they had been so good to us. From Bogota it was a 25 hour bus ride to Ecuador which really wasn't too bad. We stayed in a little town, Otavalo, in a valley surrounded by mountains. It was full of Indians where all the men wore their long black hair tied back in a braid down their backs, with a bowler hat on top. The women also had the same jet-black hair and wore lots of beads. Quito, the main city of Ecuador was a typical Spanish-style town set on top of a mountain. We preferred to stay in the old part of the town where the streets were very steep and hard to climb. We met many people there and had a great time.

Peru is a very different country [from] Ecuador. All along the coast is a hot and barren desert. We travelled through it by bus which was another very long trip. The city is extremely poor but exciting. We had some very memorable times there.

We also got letters from home, which as you would know, was great.

We went to Machu Picchu. The Inca ruins are unbelievable. We felt as if we were on top of the world. The scenery was magnificent. We climbed to the top of a mountain which overlooks the ruins. Not many people do this because it is such a hard climb but it was worth it! We could see for miles into deep valleys with huge waterfalls that went up into the clouds. We had to drag ourselves away back to Cuzco then caught a train to Arequipa. While we were in Peru a war broke out on the northern border of Ecuador. It was exciting, not scary, watching it on the news and reading about it, as well as seeing the people of Peru react to it.

Writing this letter has been great for me as it brought many memories back. I long to go back there. I am missing the travel and meeting people and seeing new places.

I am very restless, and I cannot wait to pack my back-pack once again and start traveling.

I hope all goes well with the photography, and seeing your mum once again. Write soon and tell me about it.

Bye
Caroline

About two or three days prior to coming home, her diary reveals, Tarry was still fussing about what to buy her father as a gift. She really wanted to bring home something special for dad. So preoccupied was she that she was unable to enjoy the effects of some cocaine she had been given to try. Eventually she bought him a beautifully woven rug from Peru. And although she had had her doubts about trying cocaine, she tried it just the same, and found the aftereffects very unpleasant. I found this scenario a touching blend of love for home and love for freedom.

The Tarry that we welcomed home was quite a different girl from the one we had so nervously farewelled eight weeks earlier. She bounced through the sliding customs door decked out from head to toe in brightly colored Mexican clothing. Silver earrings dangled from her ears. Her feet were bound in leather strips and thongs, and above them rose the shapely brown, but ever so hairy, legs. Swishing around her legs was a glorious green-colored cotton skirt that matched the color of her eyes. There was a narrowly woven, colored anklet tied above each foot and right wrist. Beads rattled and twinkled around her neck, and down the front of the peasant blouse, little embroidered purses dangled from silken cords. Over this she wore a short, cropped, brightly colored, coarsely woven cotton waistcoat embroidered with tiny mirrors. Her hair had grown very long and curly, and sitting on top of this mop was a black straight-brimmed peasant's hat. I couldn't believe my eyes. She looked really beautiful, stunning actually, but so very, very different.

She prattled on all the way home in the car. She couldn't get over the affluent lifestyle she deemed us to lead. The fridge, for example, delighted her – so full of good things, especially milk, orange juice and fruit, all so fresh and abundant. She could not believe that she had always taken these creature comforts for granted. It was clear that this also offended her sense of justice, such as it was at the time.

Tarry, as always, voiced her opinions, and seemed to think that the rest of us would not understand because we had not been in South America. We did understand her though, but not to the extent that we felt compelled to change our lifestyle, as she did. As it would not be easy for her to live a frugal gypsy lifestyle while at home with her parents, I knew that it would not be long before she moved out. This she did quite soon, and with our blessing. She had to do what she believed to be the right thing. And Tarry knew that the front door would always be open for her here at Kew.

Although Tarry was the first to move out of home, it was not long before the others did too. They moved close to Melbourne University where three of them were students: Kristen doing a bachelor of science and education degree; Jamie, medicine; and Margie, arts/law.

As with many of our friends who faced the empty nest syndrome with their children, our turn had come to deal with this situation. Strangely enough the kids were home more often than not. They were becoming very interesting, mature and well-informed young adults. They were great friends to each other and to us, and still are. We loved having their company. An especially welcome occurrence was the separate visits we received from their friends, their wonderful friends from childhood days. Our doors are still open, and, I am very happy to say, still frequently have a number of these friends marching through them.

When Tarry moved out, she bundled her belongings onto the roof-racks of her brother's car and bolted off to settle into a small house in Balwyn, only 10 minutes away, but far enough to maintain her precious independence. She shared this house with two other girls, one of whom was part of the South American travel contingent. She returned to her old job of sandwich-making and waitressing, and settled down to work hard to save up for her next overseas trip. She kept up with all her friends and we saw her often. She was always a pleasure to have around us. "Howdies, Ma," she would call to me as she came through the laundry door and into the kitchen.Tarry enjoyed great popularity and had many interests and friends. Her health was tip-top and altogether her life was quite normal and very happy. I was not at all concerned about her, and felt I had no reason to be. After all, mothers can't expect to know every detail of their children's personal lives, if, as in some cases, they know anything at all.

Tarry celebrated her 21st birthday here at home on January 23, 1982. It was a small, happy poolside gathering of family and friends all casually attired for a hot summer's day. A costly large party was not even considered, as Tarry preferred to have a cheque. When added to her other earnings, this money financed her next trip, this time starting in Paris. She flew off, on her own once again, on September 20 of that year.

We saw her off quite happily, particularly as she had everything well planned, and was to stay for a while with Frank's niece and her husband, who were living in Paris at that time. On the previous day, Tarry's friends and I had sat on the windowsill of her large and beautiful bedroom at Kew while we watched her carefully pack everything she would need into neat bundles, and then place them in her backpack in the order in which they would be required during the journey. As she packed away each item, she would call out what it was and we would tick it off the list. We were all so excited for her. I was longing to travel, too. I think the travel bug had bitten all our itchy feet.

Tarry threw herself body and soul into this European trip. She met friends in Paris, as planned, and they moved on through France, then down through Spain to Portugal, Morocco and Algeria, leading a very leisurely, gypsy-like life as they meandered along from here to there for nearly eight months.

Her closely written letters and postcards arrived from time to time and, like her phone calls (though infrequent), were always a joy to receive. Each card and letter was amazingly detailed, complete with tiny sketches of people and scenes that had particularly appealed to her. Her powers of description were vivid, animated and passionate. She was totally in love with life, it seemed, and she happily shared that news with those of us left at home.

Tarry also kept a journal of these travels. In it she recorded her newest experience, which was to strike real terror into my heart when I learnt of it. This experience was trying heroin in Morocco and Spain, where supplies of this drug were plentiful, and as far as I could gather, the laws regarding any kind of drug use seemed rather slack.

Tarry said it was an incredible experience. She quite openly admitted to "giving it a go" but she felt it was too dangerous to use too often as that involved the possibility of becoming addicted. She then dismissed it as yet another of life's experiences. But I fear much damage had already been done. She apparently had shared a needle, or needles, with her Spanish friends, and they did not know then, nor did we, that this was another method by which HIV/AIDS was acquired or transmitted. So that, as well as her earlier relationship with a bisexual man, had surely sealed our Tarry's fate. Her date with death had been confirmed.

I met some of Tarry's Spanish friends in Spain in 1985. They were delightful young people. I am afraid that by now, like Tarry, many of them could also be dead, or very ill. I could find out, but I dare not. I couldn't bear the pain of knowing their fate.

She was away for Christmas, but she was safe with friends in Guernica. She stayed with the family of a wonderful Basque priest friend of ours whose ministry was here in Melbourne. This family greeted her with open arms, although I heard they were a bit mystified by her appearance. The dreadlocks were in full flight around her head, she was rather shabbily dressed and very tired from her rough-and-ready gypsy lifestyle.

She was beside herself with joy to be embraced by a real family once again. Tarry had by this time learned to speak Spanish quite fluently and the advantage of being able to speak enough Spanish made everyone comfortable to be with her. She loved sharing the family's Christmas traditions, especially the unique celebration of the feast of the Epiphany on January 6, 1983. The three wise kings arrived by train into Guernica and set off on camels in a swirling mist of dry ice, distributing gifts to the children of this poor but beautiful old town. Well, beautiful until it was bombed during the Spanish Civil War.

June 1983

Anouck,

I suppose you must be wondering what happened to me.

The reason why I haven't written is because I had my pack stolen in Spain, including your address. I was only in Valencia a couple of days when everything was taken. Luckily I always keep my money and passport on me.

Apart from that I had a fantastic time in Spain and by the end of three months I could speak Spanish and understand it really well. For New Year's Eve there were 14 of us in a house in Guernica where we had the traditional ten-course meal (did I feel ill afterwards!). At 12 o'clock we turned on the T.V. which was showing the Plaza Mayor and the clock. On each stroke of 12 we had to eat a raisin.

This is done every New Year's Eve. It is meant to bring good luck for the year.
Afterwards we went to disco and bars till morning.
I went to a Carnival in Cadiz where all the people packed the streets
from 7:00 pm Saturday night until Monday morning, all in
fancy dress and crazy make-up. So as you can tell Spain was like one
big fiesta.
From Spain I went to Portugal which was completely crazy and wild,
spending most of the time in the south. I was in a town call Portimao
where I lived with a Portuguese guy.
We had a lot of fun together but he was addicted to heroin. It eventually
turned bad, and I left for Italy.
The reason I am in Italy is because mum has come over for two months,
studying Italian in Florence for one and afterwards going to Paris and
England. When we are in Paris I will pop in and say hello.
Hope you are well and your work is going O.K. See you in a few weeks.

Love Caroline

For some weeks before Christmas of 1982 I had been trying to coax
Frank into allowing me to travel to Italy to continue studying Italian
language at a school in Florence. I also worked out that this would be a
good way of catching up with Tarry again, for she had no plans to
return home in the foreseeable future. Frank agreed to this and I was so
happy to make plans for what I called my long service leave. I booked in
at the school recommended to me and made the necessary arrangements
for the flight and for accommodation in Rome and Florence.

A very well-traveled friend of mine suggested she might come with
me, and I was very pleased to have her company. She knew Italy, having
stayed there often, and was well acquainted with the European
lifestyle. When I made contact with Tarry, she seemed delighted at the
prospect of spending time with me, and I was really excited to be seeing her again after almost eight months. My friend and I flew off to
Rome, arriving there on May 29, a day and date of intense sorrow for us
10 years later.

During our long flight, I had mentally rehearsed my reunion with my beautiful, bouncy daughter. I could hardly wait to see her. However, when we emerged from customs at the Rome airport, I just couldn't believe my eyes. I could barely contain my shock at the sight Tarry presented as she came towards me.

At first I didn't recognize Tarry; she looked shocking. She was in filthy, dirty jeans and T-shirt, her complexion was muddy, her hair matted and dull and her eyes bleary and tearful. She was bent over with the weight of her backpack. She released the pack and fell into my arms totally exhausted. She had been on the road for three days, she said, in order to meet our flight, and had slept on a bench in the airport lounge that past night.

My traveling companion was marvelous. She greeted Tarry warmly, showing no shocked surprise at all. She had known Tarry as an acquaintance of her daughters when at school. She kindly gave the two of us some time to get used to the idea of being together again before we all headed off to the hotel. Before too long, though, we were hurtling along the chaotic road to Rome in a taxi that took us to the very pleasant hotel at which we had reservations for two nights before leaving for Florence. By this time I had recovered from the initial shock of Tarry's appearance and we became engrossed in the joy of reunion.

The reception area of the hotel was bustling with elegantly attired guests and not an eyebrow was raised at the ill-assorted trio that arrived at the desk to check in. Tarry and I shared a beautiful room with a view of the Spanish Steps. First up, Tarry was totally immersed in a deep hot bath for a long soak, scrub and a hair wash. Meanwhile, any item of her clothing that seemed able to stand up on its own was ditched by me into a garbage receptacle outside the hotel.

Once dressed in my jeans and white shirt and a pair of white sneakers, Tarry looked fine again, but I thought a thorough medical check-up would be wise. Tarry agreed to this, and thanks to the great kindness of a Jesuit friend of ours, who lived, worked and taught at the Gregorian University in Rome, arrangements were made for Tarry to be examined at the American Hospital.

We were collected from the hotel at 8:00 am and taken across town to the hospital. Fortunately, Tarry was given the "all clear." All she needed, it seemed, was to be with her mum for a while, along with lashings of love, reassurance, good food and accommodation. This would be no trouble at all to provide, as of course I would have done anything for her to keep her well. She responded to my care very quickly.

The holiday could now begin, and it did, in great style. The three of us headed down the Spanish Steps to the Via Condotti. We rediscovered the glorious St Peters, the Vatican Museum, the Sistine Chapel, and other attractions of Rome that my friend and our dear Jesuit friend knew so well. We had a celebratory dinner that evening at Il Rampe, a restaurant at the bottom of the Spanish Steps. Next morning, we rented a little Ritmo car, piled the luggage in, and after a few false starts in the bewildering Roman traffic, we headed off to Florence.

For the next few weeks Florence was to be home for us. The school itself was rather daunting but my friend Lorraine and I battled on with the studying, and had much more fun with Tarry after hours. Not once did the mature aged students play truant, as it was very interesting to meet and try to converse with other students from many countries. Most of the students, though, seemed to be Swiss-German and spoke little or no English.

Tarry would potter around the galleries, and even met up with some friends from home, and then we would all get together for meals and shopping and to drive to beautiful places like Lake Como on "il weekend." It was absolute magic, and Tarry blossomed. Her beauty, vim and vigor and enthusiasm had returned, and we revelled in each other's company, more like sisters than mother and daughter.

Tarry and I flew to Paris for a week, then London, then back to France, and each and every day was pure joy for both of us. Not once did a cross word pass between us, and Tarry showed no signs of restlessness or boredom from being just with me. She often spoke with great affection of her friends in Spain. She was going to meet them again after she had farewelled me at Orly Airport in Paris on July 28.

It had all been wonderful, and I was pleased that although I could enjoy that time of freedom from home and responsibilities, I was also excited at the prospect of being reunited with Frank again. There really is no place like home. I was secretly hoping that Tarry might feel the same way, change her mind and come home with me. But that was too much to hope for.

A week after I arrived home, Kristen and a friend left for an organized tour of England and Europe. She was to meet up with Tarry in Barcelona. This meeting did not eventuate, which dismayed and dis-appointed Kristen very much and worried us to some extent, also. We didn't hear from Tarry as frequently now. She was totally caught up in the company of her Spanish friends, and had fallen in love as well. That in itself would have accounted for her failure to meet up with Kristen. Being in love obliterates just about everything else, especially in the first flush of a romance.

It was during this time in Melbourne that there was a lot of talk about Tarry and her travels, which to many seemed unconventional. I don't know why. After all, she was not the only young traveler to have ven-tured off the beaten track. The gossips' hot-line was very busy, however.

The most upsetting incident for me was a conversation I overheard at our 25th wedding anniversary party, which the children held for us at Portsea on January 10, 1984. Two of the guests, who always kept themselves very busy minding everyone's business, and not their own, were saying to each other: "What a pity the only one missing is Caroline. Of course, she's on drugs, you know. That's why she hasn't come home."

I was absolutely shattered. From that moment the night for me was ruined. I was furious and rang one of these guests the following morning to say how enraged I was. This lady defended herself by saying that absolutely everyone knew that Tarry was on drugs. Everyone except her family, of course.

Five weeks later, on February 19, Tarry arrived home looking the picture of good health and happiness. She had been overseas for 18 months. I told her what was being said about her, and she laughed this off. She admitted that she had tried a few things, told a few friends, and, as she said, "Well, you know what Melbourne is like, so and so is always first with an exaggerated form of the latest." Quite right. So I put that behind me.

May 1984

Hi Anouck,

Well here I am back home and it feels a little weird.
A lot of things have changed, some for the better and some for the not so
good, but overall its exciting seeing everyone again.
Everything had got quite out of control over here in the last few months
that I was away. There were all sorts of rumors going around that I was
heavily involved in drugs, not only with hash but heroin as well!!
If only people would mind their own business life would be much easier.
I still don't know what I want to do, so I'll settle for doing nothing
at the moment.
Well, so much for me. How are you? How's Serge and your work?
Lots of questions, but am hoping for lots of answers.
Take care.

Love Caroline
P.S. Will send a photo in next letter.

Once home, Tarry was full of stories of Spain and her Spanish boyfriend, who lived in Gijon on the north coast of Spain. She was sad to leave him, but felt she had to. She wanted to be home again, for a while at least, although not at Kew.

Soon after arriving home, Tarry moved into a type of commune in Carlton. Apparently this quite attractive building had once been a convent, with a community of nuns. The accommodation there was a series of rabbit-warren rooms running up and down little flights of stairs, all haphazardly arranged around a large living room with very basic kitchen and bathroom facilities. Tarry was very excited about her new home, and after she settled herself and her belongings into her little room, she invited me around for a visit.

I nearly fainted when I saw the setup, not to mention the other residents, who all looked at me as though I was a visitor from another world. Well, that was fair enough. I thought the same way about them. They seemed to me to be unfriendly, sloppy and perhaps stoned as well. I suppose Tarry considered these living arrangements to be the closest resemblance to her lifestyle in Spain. It looked to me like the fringe of the underworld. But it was Tarry's decision and her life, and she was so happy and proud to show me around her new dwelling place. I couldn't help but enthuse along with her. I told her how clever she was to find somewhere so different, friendly, light and airy to live. It was so close to the city and her workplace too.

After the tour of inspection and a cup of tea, I was introduced to a tall, blond Adonis, dressed in a loose tie-dyed cheesecloth shirt and washed-out pink baggy cotton pants with drawstrings around the waist and ankles. He had beads around his neck, and a headband of tiny wooden beads held back his long blond hair. This was the new boyfriend, and the only one she would be with again, for better or worse. I sensed the latter. They were very taken with each other, and their relationship was to last a long time.

In 1985, after consulting once more with Frank, a trip to Spain was planned. Tarry had saved up her money again and, by living frugally, had enough money to resume her travels. This time I asked if I would be able to come too. She was thrilled with the idea and wrote to her French friend about it.

July 1985

Dear Anouck,
In five weeks time I am going back to Spain! My mother has
always wanted to see Spain so she asked me to go with her and show
her around. We are only going for five weeks.
One week in London and four in Spain. We are meeting my brother,
younger sisters and friends and hiring a car to drive around Spain.
Because we have so short a time I won't be able to visit you in Paris
which I would love.
I enjoyed your last letter. It sounds as though you are enjoying life
and you are happy (still)?

Next time I am moving into a lovely small cottage tucked away
in a quiet street. It will be a welcome change.
Hope you are well and happy.

ALWAYS Caroline XX

As it turned out, there were to be eight of us. Dominique was in Greece; Jamie, who had been working in a hospital in New Zealand, was due for a few weeks holiday; Margie was free and able to come along; and my sister agreed to join us as well. Two more of the children's friends made up the party. Frank wasn't able to take the time off, but didn't mind paying for me, and Kristen agreed to look after her dad, so it was with enormous excitement and joy that this memorable trip was planned.

And there are no prizes for guessing who did all the organizing of the Spanish part of the adventure. Tarry pored over maps choosing locations, towns, cities and villages and the best way to follow the path she chose was to hire a mini-bus, working out the safest routes but not the main highways. Tarry planned the most amazing, carefully drawn-up itinerary.

We left Melbourne on Saturday, August 3, 1985. After a week in a London flat, Tarry and Jamie flew off to Madrid, picked up the mini-bus and drove to Bilbao, where we all met up at the airport. Thereafter our adventures began. The Basque separatists were busy throwing bombs here and there in their efforts to attain their independence, but luckily for us we were not in the wrong places at the wrong time and were spared any dangerous situations. We drove right through the Basque country, camping here and there along the way. We joined in the most wonderful festivals, the most memorable of which was in Bermeo, a tiny fishing village where we were made most welcome.

We spent a magic night in Bermeo high up on the mountains overlooking the wild and crashing seas of the Bay of Biscay. Thanks to Tarry and her ability to speak Spanish, we joined a group of wonderful young men and women all dressed in pale blue cotton shorts and overalls with metal soup ladles hanging around their necks. They were stirring huge black iron pots filled with a delicious fish stew. They were singing and dancing and invited us to join them. They explained to us, through Tarry, that this was a festival which was held each year to celebrate their liberation from the oppression of the days of the Franco reign of terror. Bermeo is very close to Guernica. We ate, sang, danced and laughed in this magical ring until daylight.

Later that day we drove further west along the coast to Gijon. This was the home town of Tarry's friend Nano, who lived with his family in a small flat in this mining seaside town. We visited Nano's warm, hospitable and loving family, with whom we spent the most wonderful day sharing food, wine, laughter and recipes. Caroline was becoming quite visibly worn out with all the interpreting for Nano's parents and me. Jamie played his guitar with the boys, and the grandchildren played happily with all of us. We exchanged gifts, as is the custom there, and in the evening we hugged them all goodbye with teary promises to return one day – each knowing, of course, that we never would.

They really loved Caroline. I simply cannot write to them to tell them she is dead. We used to exchange Christmas cards, but we don't anymore. Perhaps the young and handsome Nano is dead, too. The thought is enough to make me cry again.

We drove south toward Madrid, camping all the way. I couldn't believe I would love this simple life so much. I had always been accustomed to five star hotels, but found this much more fun. It was the company, of course. Frank would never have survived such conditions. I couldn't do it now, either, for I am older, tire easily and like to be spoiled when I travel.

We were heading for Segovia, along a route that avoided heavy transports and lorries, but was still rather hazardous. Jamie was driving and Tarry was the navigator, and by the time we reached Segovia, they were both thoroughly exhausted, especially Tarry, who had in fact quite suddenly become very ill.

A hotel near the famous aqueduct had the vacancy sign up, so we booked in there for the night. Tarry had a screaming headache, high temperature, nausea, backache and joint pains. The onset was very sudden and severe. We tucked her into bed and Jamie set about examining her carefully. He was quite a competent and knowledgeable fourth year medical student, near to the completion of his course, so he was adequately qualified to decide what was wrong with Tarry. We thought it would be too distressing for her to face the hassles of doctors in a hospital where the English language could be a problem, and Tarry was in no condition to be interpreting.

Jamie couldn't find anything specific, so he quite rightly diagnosed a reaction to complete emotional and physical exhaustion, and we all agreed, including Tarry, that this must be the case. Three years later, we would be inclined to believe that it was the hitherto dormant HIV virus beginning to stir into life in Tarry's body. This perhaps was the first manifestation of its ugly and frightening presence. Had a blood test been done even at that time nothing related to AIDS may have shown up. The insidious reign of terror had begun.

After my sister, Maria, and Margie had helped Tarry take a soothing bath and given her some Panadol and lots of mineral water to drink, I sat beside her bed stroking her hot, dry forehead until she slept. How often I was to do this in the years to come. Only, this time, I wasn't really worried.

Tarry slept well and deeply, and had made a remarkable recovery by the following morning, so we drove on again toward Madrid. During this leg of the journey Tarry dozed on and off while the rest of us organized the meals, and navigation was taken in turns, following Tarry's previously written instructions and maps.

Tarry showed no further signs of illness during this trip. Her flagging spirits began to lift again, to soar actually, as she whizzed us around all the sights and delights of Madrid. We visited the weekly Rastro market, where Tarry bargained in Spanish for goods, and bought clothing, keepsakes and gifts and showed us how to do the same.

She led us to the Plaza Mayor in the early evenings, where we gathered with many others around little wrought-iron tables to drink sangria, eat tapas and baby lamb, and listen to magnificent musicians playing guitars and pianos. They were usually in little groups and had a solo instrument or voice. The weather was warm and darkness did not descend until about 10:00 pm.

Sometimes Jamie would bring along his guitar to play, as he had on the sea wall in Bermeo, or as he leant against a eucalypt in the camping grounds. He usually gathered a very interested audience around him, especially when he played Asturias.

Tarry took us to the magnificent Prado Museo, filled with stunning works of art. Along with Margie, Tarry was the gallery guide for us, both having studied art attentively for many years. Their favorites were among the Goya collection. Some of the Goyas gave Margie horrific nightmares, but she loved them just the same.

After the Prado, we crossed a little street to a small gallery which at that time housed Picasso's "Guernica." Its ferocity and anguish reduced me to tears. It was sensational. It was displayed across one wall of an hermetically sealed glass room, closely guarded by armed uniformed women of Wagnerian proportions. Tarry carefully explained each segment of this painting to us. She did this so clearly, patiently and emotionally that she attracted the attention of other English-speaking tourists, who listened closely to what she had to say. I was so proud of her, and amazed at her knowledge.

Maria had left for Italy by train on the previous day. Tarry guided her to the station and saw her onto the train to Rome, where she would stay with friends, then go on to other friends in Paris. We would hopefully all meet up again at Heathrow Airport Lounge on September 5 for the flight home to Melbourne.

Tarry was still managing all our daily adventures in Spain. We drove from Madrid as far south as Granada, camping along the way at night. The weather was still delightfully warm and clear. It was heaven drifting happily along from one delight to the next. The most beautiful place of all was the Allhambra on the hills just outside Granada, under whose spell we all certainly fell, just as the old song says. Tarry knew the right time to arrive at the Allhambra and Generalife gates to obtain the cheapest possible sightseeing tickets. She was very adept at this and was always extremely cheerful. The locals loved her, or it seemed to me that they at least admired her sparkling, mischievous eyes.

Then it was time to return to Madrid. We reluctantly left the two young extras to find their way to Morocco. I was worried about this, but there was nothing we could do to prevent them going. As planned, we met Maria in London and we flew home together, leaving

Dominique and Jamie to continue their travels. Jamie sold his surfboard in Madrid to a highly delighted youngster.

Maria, Margie, Tarry and I arrived home on Saturday, September 7, 1985. I can honestly say that it was the most memorable and magical holiday of my life. Frank was bowled over by our stories of all our adventures. I felt like a young girl once more, although I aged a bit when the bills came in. Even camping didn't lighten the financial burden by many pesetas, and of course I had to shop when I could, especially in Madrid.

Only nine months later Tarry and Margie flew off to China and Tibet. Tarry had had no further illness, apart from the occasional cold, since her return from Spain. We still had no reason to suspect that she was harboring any sort of illness at all. So the appropriate health certificates and visas were carefully packed into their luggage, courtesy of Tarry. The two sisters left together at noon on May 31, 1986, their first port of call Hong Kong.

They called us reverse charges from Hong Kong on Sunday, June 1. This was the first day of winter in Australia and seven years later would be a day of great sadness for the family. Margie had suddenly developed severe colic and diarrhea and Tarry's super efficiency had come unstuck in the medication department of their travel packs. In order to make some room in their backpack, Tarry had emptied every pill from every bottle into one large bottle so they were unable to identify which pill did what. These assorted pills and tablets were for diarrhoea, constipation, nausea and vomiting, the type of ailments one can encounter while traveling.

Frank had to get out his copy of MIMS, a large pharmaceutical dictionary which lists and identifies all medications by color, shape, size, dosage and use, and manufacturing logos. After about one hour, and a million phone call dollars later, all pills had been sorted out and identified, and Margie's medication was ready to go into action. What a fiasco. And what strange irony that within two years, in the effort to keep AIDS illnesses from making their attack, Tarry would be taking almost as many pills as the entire contents of that bottle on a daily basis, all of which would become as familiar to her as the back of her hand.

Margie and Caroline both kept closely written and very descriptive journals of each day's activities, and later it was very interesting to read and compare their differing observations of the same situations.

December 1986

Dear Anouck,
I sent a post card to you from Lhasa, Tibet. I hope you received
it as I did not remember how to spell your surname. My sister, Margie,
whom I was traveling with in China went on to Europe.
I gave her your address.
In all I spent five months traveling around China and Tibet.
Language was bit of problem but manageable. I preferred Tibet
to China as the people are more easy-going and have a better ability of
communicating non-verbally than the Chinese.
In northern China, particularly Inner Mongolia, the people stop and stare
without a smile or any effort to acknowledge the fact that you are also a
human being, not a rare animal.
In contrast, the Tibetan people are very warm and friendly.
Communication carried out by touch of hands and smiles.
Lhasa is a very special place. Even though their God-King, the
Dalai Lama is no longer there, Lhasa and its great temples is still very
much a Mecca for this very devoted race. There are   people who have
prostrated 2,000 kilometers to eventually arrive in Lhasa.
What I mean by Prostrate is that they stretch themselves out flat on the
ground, then rise and walk to where their outstretched hands were and
once again fall to the ground. A hell of a way to travel!!
The population of Lhasa at any time consists mainly of these and other
people who have made similar long journeys.
We were very lucky to be able to stay with a Tibetan family in
a spare room that held views of the whole town of Lhasa,
the Potala (the Dalai Lama residence) and the surrounding mountains.
They were a fantastic family and it was very good of them to let us stay,

for if the Chinese found out it would of [sic] cost them almost a year's wages in fines.

We did a lot of traveling into remote areas of Tibet which was an unforgettable experience. At times [we] walked along with the Nomads, the Golok people, very wild and free, reflecting the very wild landscape they live in. They always had a small herd of yaks, amazing animals, prehistoric and brutal in appearance, but very gentle in nature. One place we went to was called Lake Nam Co at 4,700 meters. I think it may be the highest named lake in the world. To get to it we had to cross a pass at 600 meters, followed by a three-day trek to a large rock, on the lakes edge, that held 14 caves belonging, at one time, to monks or hermits. The only people to be found in this extraordinary world were the Golok people and their yaks and goats. There were also wild horses, wolves and enormous ravens, the size of a dog. No scrub or tree to be found except around the caves where we found edible nettles which were cooked over a dried yak dung fire. We stayed and walked in that wild world for ten days, which will always remain a very vivid memory.

I hitched out of Tibet on the south eastern road which took four weeks to cover 2,000 kilometers. We had to cross landslides (very scary), flooded rivers, walk another 120 kilometers, cross high passes and more wild wide rivers like Mekong and the Yellow River. It was hard going at times, but great fun.

Actually it is illegal for foreigners to travel anywhere in Tibet apart from Lhasa and two other large towns. This added to the adventure of it all. So you see I haven't forgotten you. Its just that it takes me a while to get around to writing. Please let me know how you are and what you are doing with your life.

Have a very Happy Xmas if you celebrate that sort of thing.

Lots of Love
from Caroline
P.S. Hope you like the hand-made paper.

Caroline was the more adventurous of the two. She would meet and deal with situations head-on – tickets for buses and trains, accommodation and money exchange, haggling her way towards a bargain every time. She could also handle the local people well. She had an innate understanding and respect for their different ways of life. She knew when to be forthright and pushy and always forged on with confidence. This was quite the opposite to the way she managed her life later on at home, where she became indecisive, insecure and hesitant. She freely admitted to this strange contrast in attitudes.

Margie, on the other hand, was a more timid traveler. She was happy to leave Tarry to deal with the more difficult areas of travel, which required nerves of steel and split-second timing. By contrast, Margie was very confident and capable and businesslike when surrounded by people, locations and things familiar to her at home. They complemented each other beautifully as traveling companions. They had always been very close friends, and were equally sensitive and gentle with family, friends and strangers. This was all mixed in with a very good measure of common sense.

One of their most memorable adventures in China, which they enjoyed equally, was their visit to Huan-Shan. This was the collective name for 72 mountain peaks which rise up in the south of the province of An-Hui. Legends surround many of these peaks and these were all recorded to some extent in their diaries seen through their different eyes.

The highest mountain peak was the one they chose to climb, and they did it. It was 18,700 feet (5,700 meters) above sea level and was referred to as the "Now I believe it peak." It was a precarious climb, although they were assisted by guides. When they reached the top, they were rewarded with incredibly beautiful views of the lower mountain summits, valleys and gorges, which they glimpsed through swirling clouds. Rock formations that resembled monkeys, birds and squirrels were explained to the girls by way of mythical stories. These rocky creatures had once been real, but were turned to stone as punishment for preferring the beauty of Huan-Shan to the beauty of their own heaven.

Another legend which greatly appealed to Tarry was that of the orchestral birds, or the Huan-Shan musicians. These were literally hundreds of birds all swooping and singing with joyous, melodic and continuous sound. These birds are said to be "celestial maidens" who came down from heaven to Huan-Shan to look for their sister who had strayed there and had fallen in love with her newly-found heaven. She had refused to leave. Her sisters also fell in love with this beautiful place. They, too, were turned into birds, doomed to live and sing there forever.

Tarry thought the birds definitely got the best end of what was supposed to be a miserable bargain. She was not a believer in the Catholic schoolgirl concept of heaven at all. In fact, Tarry's strongest belief regarding life after death was reincarnation. She could be really amusing about this.

On one occasion I remember bursting into laughter when she suggested that in one of her previous lives she must have been her father's mother, a very kind and good mother, perfect in every way. This explained why Frank was always so solicitous of her well-being, both physical and mental, ever ready to support her with love and tenderness. His demonstration of all these qualities during her distressing, frightening years of AIDS served to strengthen this belief of Tarry's.

It was during her travels in China and Tibet, some time of which was spent with Buddhists and Tibetan monks, that Tarry's interest in, and love of, eastern philosophies was to grow and be nurtured in her. Her ability to find a balance between eastern and western beliefs would be a great source of spiritual strength when the end of her life drew near. After the monumental climb up and down the mountain at Huan-Shan, the girls were befriended by a Chinese doctor. He practiced both eastern and western medicine. He gave each of them a massage at his clinic, and after massaging Tarry, he suggested that her liver should be more closely examined and tested when she returned home. Perhaps this was another early indication of the AIDS virus getting down to the business of destroying her auto-immune system.

On and on they trekked, traveling and camping with a group of young people and some nomads and their families, with whom they shared their food and equipment. They even indulged in yak-butter tea, which they found to be quite palatable after a few attempts in which they had to fight down the nausea. It was impolite to refuse this hospitality.

Margie had made plans to travel from Hong Kong to Europe, which she did, but Caroline continued upon her oriental journey. However, she became ill with jaundice and fever, apparently after eating tainted food, and was unable to continue the rough and arduous way of life. She sought help at a very makeshift and ill-equipped hospital, where it seemed that the sole aim of the staff was to separate Tarry from her money while at the same time administering very haphazard and crude medical and nursing care. As patients were not given the freedom to discharge themselves from hospital as they are in Australia and most other countries, a plan had to be devised to help Tarry escape from this hospital.

Two young German men who had been traveling with her would visit each day, bringing with them selections of palatable food for Tarry to try to eat. At the same time they plotted her escape from the hospital. After each visit, they took some of Tarry's belongings away with them, until after a week they had spirited away all her possessions. They used her passport (God knows how) and money to purchase an airline ticket for her return home. They also bought a train ticket to some remote place for Tarry to leave in her bedside table. This was done to put the hospital authorities off the trail once they had discovered Tarry had gone.

Early on the morning of her planned escape, Tarry picked up her towel to go to the bathroom, walked out of the hospital door and into a taxi, where her friends were waiting for her with her backpack, passport, airline ticket and suitable clothes to wear for her flight home. They took her to the airport and saw her safely into the departure lounge.

An incredible story of daring, we all thought, and I am sure it lost nothing in the telling.

This was the last time that Tarry would ever travel outside Australia. Her adventurous days were now over, for her HIV status would be diagnosed just over a year later, a diagnosis she would keep to herself until that horrendous day in October 1988. Tarry arrived home on October 28, 1986. We were all absolutely agog when she told us of her hospital experience and her daredevil method of escaping. We actually bragged about all her adventures, but Frank's reaction was rather more cautious. He immediately carried out a series of blood tests, which thankfully showed all clear. All clear! How wrong that would prove to be.

The tests showed that there was no residual liver damage, and that everything else indicated that the illness had been hepatitis A, not B. At this time the more sinister hepatitis C had only been vaguely referred to in the current medical journals, so was not considered in Tarry's tests, nor was HIV/AIDS.

Soon Tarry was very well again and had resumed her hard-working life at her old job. Life in the Carlton Convent had been exchanged for other accommodation in a house in Brunswick, with the blond-haired boyfriend still, and three others. Tarry's plan now was to save up for a prolonged trip to India, after which, she was to tell me, she hoped to settle down. Marriage and longed-for children were her ultimate, and hopefully, her most fulfilling goal. Sadly none of these plans would ever be realized.

Chapter 8

ᴕ

A Lull in the Storm

My story now reverts to Monday, March 9, 1991, as our plane approached San Francisco airport for touchdown at 3:35 pm local time. We had left Melbourne on the same calendar date at 1.30 pm local time.

I pulled myself out of my reveries and forward on to 1991, skipping over the three intervening years of shock and grief. Now was the time for happiness, for we were about to land in San Francisco. Our own adventures were beginning and my memories of Tarry's happy traveling were carefully stowed away in my head and heart for future reference.

We checked into our hotel and, as advised by the medical staff at Fairfield Hospital, telephoned the chief-of-staff in the AIDS unit for an appointment. We had a letter of introduction with us but we learned that the doctor concerned had received an urgent call elsewhere. So an appointment was made for the following morning with another member of this unit. We felt very pleased that one of our prime reasons for coming to America was soon to be justified. In eager anticipation of the next day, we went to bed early to have a complete rest.

Our first day was spent at San Francisco General Hospital, as we had planned. It was a grim experience. The hospital building was gray, cold, austere and unfriendly. We followed what seemed to be miles of painted lines around corridors, and in and out of lifts, which finally led us to the AIDS department. This in itself was a real fright. We caught the occasional glimpse of a gaunt-faced patient behind a little glass pane in a solid door. It all seemed so isolated and lonely, and bare of any color and warmth. I had never encountered such an atmosphere of hopelessness in a hospital before.

No one seemed at all interested in being helpful to us foreigners. We finally found ourselves in a cluttered sort of conference room, with a big oval table almost filling it from wall to wall. Clutching Tarry's history, Frank and I wedged ourselves into the straight-backed chairs. We waited interminably for the consulting doctor. Although we had made an appointment, the doctor failed to arrive. Instead, we were met by someone else, who gave Tarry's history a cursory glance up and down, then looked at us rather doubtfully. The hospital had very little experience of females with AIDS, the woman remarked. Really there was nothing she could tell us that we didn't already know.

That, of course, was of no help at all, seeing as we didn't know anything much to begin with. We left the hospital feeling really defeated and downhearted. Our letter of introduction from Fairfield Hospital had not produced the results we had hoped for. We were somewhat cheered, though, to realize that when it comes to dealing with AIDS, Fairfield must be as good a hospital as anywhere in the world, if the San Francisco General Hospital was anything to go by. This experience served to strengthen our sense of security in Fairfield Hospital, the old, familiar and extremely competent infectious diseases hospital back home in Melbourne. *Please God, keep that wonderful place functioning for ever, out of the clutches of other institutions which might want to swallow up their facilities, and fragment the care of AIDS patients.* On our arrival back at the beautiful Westin Saint Francis Hotel, we agreed then and there to put all AIDS business to one side. With that decided, we then managed to have a really wonderful holiday.

San Francisco was superb, but the main attraction for us was Margie in Washington DC. When we arrived at the airport, she was waiting there for us with a stretch limousine ready to transport us to our hotel. I couldn't believe such luxury.

We were so excited to see Margie again. She looked the epitome of young American style, elegant and confident. She was so chic and so very beautiful, warm and loving. I shed a few tears as we wrapped each other up in a big bear hug. At the hotel, the three of us sat by the fire having a light supper. We talked and talked. It was like a beautiful dream. We were happier than we had been for such a long time.

Margie's special man arrived from Australia two days later. They announced their engagement that evening. It was such a joyous occasion, and so romantic. We rang home. Tarry answered the phone with shrieks of enthusiasm. It was first-hand news for her, but not for Dominique, who had tried the engagement ring on for size some weeks earlier.

We all had our collective fingers crossed that Tarry would stay well, and still be with us for Margie's wedding, which was planned for March 1992, just 12 months away. It had become such a habit with me when any plans were made for the future always to wonder what Tarry's state of health would be. She was always first to be considered in my mind, and I am sure the others must have been irritated by this at times. I just couldn't help myself. This was quite natural, I suppose.

From Washington the four of us flew to Boston, where we were lucky enough to find the perfect wedding dress for Margie. It was just beautiful, exquisitely embroidered with the finest cream French lace and we bought it right then. We hired a car and meandered through the glorious beauty of New England in spring. It was extremely relaxing and interesting, especially as we came to know Margie's fiance Peter better. If travelers can get along well together while on the road, they'll be happy with each other under any circumstances.

We spent four wonderful days in New York, kissed our Margie and Peter goodbye, and having lit yet another candle for Tarry in St Patrick's Cathedral, flew off to England.

This trip to England was to be a kind of pilgrimage for Frank. He would visit Oxford, the university city of his dreams, and the home of Cardinal John Henry Newman. Cardinal Newman was an eminent churchman of the Victorian era. For more than 50 years Frank had studied this great man and his writings very closely, and he had enormous admiration for him.

We arrived in Oxford with two very close friends from Australia. We would be traveling with them for the last few weeks of our holiday. They were marvelous company, and entered into the spirit of the search for Cardinal Newman's cottages at Littlemore with great enthusiasm.

Once the search was commenced, we came across the signpost to Littlemore quite suddenly. Frank was driving carefully along the road leading out of Oxford when he braked, reversed up the road, and turned right. There in front of us were the cottages, with Cardinal Newman's coat of arms *cor ad cor loquitur* (heart speaks to heart) over one of the front doors. Frank was beside himself, a most unusual state for him, as unlike his wife, he is not given to displays of emotion. We lit candles in the adjacent church, and I could see Frank praying earnestly to Cardinal Newman, who is presently a candidate for canonization.

In order to be canonized, the candidate must perform a certain number of miracles which can be attributed solely to the intercession of the said candidate. This ritual is peculiar to the Roman Catholic Church, and I know that Frank had prayed every day since October 12, 1988, for Cardinal Newman's intervention on Caroline's behalf. Frank is a true scholar and academic, and a devout but realistic Catholic. His supplication to Cardinal Newman would have been a deeply spiritual one.

Personally I have trouble understanding this type of prayer. I just felt that if John Henry Newman wanted to become a saint, well, here was his big chance. He could start his miracles by curing Caroline. But that was over-simplifying things, so I just said, "Please, please, do something, if you can," lit another candle and left it at that.

I have to admit that, in a way, my prayer was answered, because contrary to all expectations, when the time came, Caroline had a wondrously peaceful and tranquil death. She had happily received the last sacraments and was enveloped in abundant love and security. It is not infrequent that AIDS patients die still raging, resentful and fearful.

Next we drove on to Birmingham to the oratory where Cardinal Newman had his private chapel, library and office. All these rooms and their contents were just as he had left them. His prie-dieu, vestments, cardinal's hat, books and violin – everything was all beautifully preserved. Frank was so happy. He derived such pleasure from absorbing the atmosphere, touching, feeling and seeing the belongings of the man whom he had for so long admired and loved. The priest in charge of the oratory, with whom Frank spoke at length, seemed amazed at the depth of Frank's knowledge of this great man. Frank knelt to pray on the little prie-dieu in the chapel, and I knew then it was mission accomplished.

After a week of light-hearted and lyrical frolicking around Ireland with our good and kindly friends, we returned to London for a week of theater, galleries and shopping for all. Our friends then left for France and we eagerly flew home to Australia, arriving on May 2.

CHAPTER 9

୬

PLOTTING A NEW COURSE

The television ad for Australia's national airline Qantas, titled "I Still Call Australia Home," appears to have considerable popular appeal, but the long haul from London's Heathrow airport to Tullamarine airport in Melbourne dampens one's feelings of exhilaration at returning home. The last six to seven hours across our own vast continent seems so interminable and the 5:00 am arrival just finished us off. Along with an undercurrent of in-flight fatigue was an uneasy feeling of uncertain hope and foreboding fear of the future.

Kristen, always so dependable, met us at the customs door at 6:00 am. She drove us home to Kew and it was so wonderful to be there and hold everyone close to us again. That evening, the family prepared and cooked a "Welcome Home" dinner, everyone's favorite, wing rib of beef. During the evening they were delighted to receive the special gifts we had brought home for them from England, Ireland and America.

It was to Tarry, though, that my gaze kept returning. I looked into her eyes, and I saw in them the edges of fear. I felt the tears spring into my own eyes. I loved her so much, but little by little she was slipping away from me. I held her tightly in my gaze for a long time. She mustn't leave us yet. Please, Tarry, don't go yet.

I looked away. I had to swallow all this pain for now and keep myself together, for there would be many times later on when to do this would be virtually impossible. I ran upstairs and got dressed up in a beautiful Italian suit, complete with silk shirt, shoes and bag to match and a stunning hat that Frank had bought for me in a very smart shop in Bond Street in London. This was to wear to Margie's wedding. I regaled the family with the exaggerated story of how the Italian boutique owner thought I was the Dottore's mistress, because of the amount of money Frank had spent on buying this outfit for me.

Tarry laughed along with the others, and the moments of tension eased. She insisted that she was, and had been, perfectly well, and that she was still very happy in Brunswick, and wished to continue living there.

Perhaps it was the prospect of the imminent arrival of yet another Melbourne winter that was frightening Tarry. She admitted as much, saying that while she wanted no further discussion about her state of health, she would like to top up the winter wardrobe. We set off on Monday morning, two days later, to do just that.

It was while she was trying clothes on in the various shops that I noticed the strange thinness had returned. She was down to a small size 8, from the adequately filled size 10 she was before we went away. Perhaps she had not been keeping to a proper diet. I decided I would say nothing about this to her.

Our Sally, as well as the Fairfield dietitian, worked out another very palatable high calorie diet for Caroline to select from during the coming winter months. I had supplied Caroline with an electric blender so that she could whip up egg-flips and thickshakes with added Sustagen whenever she wished. But that was where the problem lay. Her appetite, for the present anyway, was not good. Fear alone was forcing her to eat, and fear is not a good aperitif.

About this time, Frank and I decided that we should arrange a meeting with Caroline's doctor. We were anxious to know exactly what the situation was regarding Caroline's present state of health and hoped to receive some sort of prognosis.

We had never actually met this doctor, although we had exchanged phone calls on the occasions when Caroline was ill. An appointment was duly made to meet this doctor on Thursday, June 13, 1991, at 2:00 pm. The doctor, a young woman, had an almost worldwide reputation for her competence in caring for AIDS patients. She had enormous demands made on her as the numbers of AIDS patients were increasing at an alarming rate. The doctor was constantly on the run from patients' bedsides, to outpatients, other hospitals, meetings, and press and TV interviews. Amazingly, she seemed to manage all these duties with calmness and common sense. I could tell what a truly wonderful person she was by the way she really seemed to care about Frank and me, and, of course, Caroline.

Frank and I were so nervous as we sat in the waiting room. God knows what we would hear. The doctor arrived, warmly welcomed us and sat down opposite us as though she had all the time in the world. Not once did she glance at her watch, look impatient or shuffle the papers around on her lap. We had her undivided attention. She told us that it was the unknown that worried her, as much as it did us. Little progress had been made in the field of finding a cure or vaccine for HIV/AIDS despite intensive research around the clock, and around the world.

However, it was considered that if Caroline were to continue keeping as well as she was now, in spite of her weight loss and the MAC, she could be expected to live for quite some time yet. We were told that Caroline was a wonderful, courageous and dignified patient who had won the admiration and the hearts of all the staff who had dealings with her. She was very pleased with the way that Caroline looked after herself. She also added that it had been an enormous advantage for Caroline to be on the receiving end of so much loving care from her family and friends. Unlike those with AIDS who had to fend for themselves when they were not in the hospital wards, she was in a very safe, nurturing environment, which hopefully would prolong her life.

The doctor then unravelled my confusion concerning all the medications and their uses and effects, and reassured me that I could confidently go ahead and plan Margie's wedding, and not Caroline's funeral. We had a bit of a grim chuckle about that.

Frank was shown the greatest respect, gentleness and courtesy. Caroline's wonderful doctor knew his frustrating dilemma of being a doctor himself and unable to help his daughter. We mentioned the possibility of importing a new drug, DDC, from New York. It was not quality controlled, nor was it officially approved by the Food and Drug Administration (FDA), but it was available if patients wanted to try it, buy it and import it independently.

Caroline was brave enough, and so eager to try anything at all that might prolong her life. So it was agreed that we could go ahead and order this new drug. When we left the doctor's room after about an hour, we felt reassured and very happy that we had established a rapport with her as people, not just as Caroline's parents at home on the other end of the telephone. We felt we could all work together now towards maintaining a safe state of health for our mutual patient, Caroline.

In July Tarry was given the opportunity to take a holiday in Byron Bay on the north coast of New South Wales with a friend of Kristen. A house and a car would be available for their use during their stay. The excitement was enormous. Tarry couldn't believe her good fortune. She could escape the Melbourne winter she dreaded so much for at least two weeks. The date of departure was Friday, July 12. Once again Tarry filled up her backpack, so happy to be including bathing suits, suntan lotion, sun hat and shorts, as well as the inevitable supply of medications. As we drove her to the airport, Tarry was singing her way along the Tullamarine freeway. I had not seen her so chortly since her earlier independent traveling days.

August 1991

Dear Anouck,
Sorry for taking so long to reply. It is just that my life seems so
unorganized. Physically I am okay but mentally I am very confused.
Trying to face reality is not easy, even a little frightening but I feel now
that it is becoming a little easier to confront.
Thank you for your letter, it made me feel good inside, not only
to realize what a special person you are, but also it pulled me up a bit.
I've spent so much time feeling sorry for myself, crying.
It's not fair, hating life and everyone around me, that for a while I lost
perspective on things. Reading about your work in Hong Kong made me
realize how fortunate I am (living in a wealthy country, security of
family etc) but how self-centered I've become. My focus of attention is
still on myself but in a more positive way which makes life less miserable
for myself, but, more importantly for those around me.
I've just come back from a wonderful holiday in Northern N.S.W.

A place called Byron Bay. A warm beautiful place where the sun shines
every day and dolphins (hundreds of them) play in the shallows.
It's a place of healing, a center for alternative life styles and ideas.
It made Melbourne seem such a dark, cold place where disease can fester.
I'm not sure if it was being there or whether it was just that
time in my life when I needed to change, but I am changing bit
by bit, beginning to realize that I can cure myself, I can live for
as long as I want, I have that power.
For so long now I have studied Eastern philosophies in a very dry
academic way, but now I am setting out to practice them.
Not just sticking to one but taking a bit from one and integrating it with
another to eventually come to an understanding of what life is all about.
I believe that by seeing clearly and having a conviction of a philosophy I
will be a bit less confused about myself. Yoga, meditation and a lot of
reading will help.
So this is what I will be doing for the rest of this year and maybe I will go
back to Byron Bay to live for a while.
That will be a difficult decision to make. It's strange that I can travel to
foreign lands and explore unknown (to me) cultures with courage and
excitement, but when it comes to situations closer to me; emotions and
thoughts, I can be so timid.
By the way I encourage you every bit of the way in your writing.
Writing, whether fiction or non-fiction is a wonderful thing to do.
It is something I wish I could do well. Do not worry about the lack of
inspiration from people around you. It is what is inside yourself that is
important. The love and inspiration from within is all you need.

All my love
Your friend from afar!
Caroline

This was the first "real holiday" she had taken without Frank and
me since AIDS had taken over her life. Those two weeks were the last

really happy days she was to spend away from home and family while she was still well. She sent postcards telling of the joy of it all, and they are still sticky-taped to the fridge door. Every day for her was filled with sun and warmth and fun.

Byron Bay is the seaside heart of Alternative Lifestyle Country. It has beautiful beaches populated by ageing hippies clinging to their halcyon days when they were the flower children of the sixties. There are young people too, seeking the "meaning of life" and aided in their search by various means, illicit or otherwise, all available at Byron Bay.

Many naturopaths, masseurs, aromatherapists, iridologists, all well-qualified in the practice of natural medicine, can also be found at Byron. Tarry sought the help of some of these practitioners and they were wonderful to her. Among them she found an old friend from school days, who introduced her to people who read her eyes, and gave her massages. They boosted her self image and confidence and, best of all, they gave her hope. Not "false hope", either. I do not believe there is such a thing as "false hope." Hope is always real and positive. Of the three cardinal virtues, Faith, Hope and Charity, Hope seems to me to be the most significant. It is harder to attain and hold on to when the odds seem stacked against having any hope at all, especially when a frightening illness like AIDS is tightening its grip.

Tarry never relinquished her hold on hope of some sort. When she realized that hope for a long life on this earth was not an option, she gradually transferred her hopes to attaining a happy life after death. It would take a long time for this switch to occur fully, though, and many angry and ferocious battles would rage within and without during the transition from one hope to the other.

Margie was due to arrive home from America the week after Tarry left for Byron Bay. There were great plans afoot for a large "welcome home" party for her, which would also be a celebration of her engagement to Peter. We were all eagerly awaiting her arrival, as most of the guests had not seen Margie for a long time, and very few friends had met her fiance.

Tarry was very pleased that she would be away for this party. She dreaded being under any form of scrutiny. I was just as pleased that she was not here, for it meant that I could proceed with all the party arrangements without having to worry about the effect it might have on her. She and Margie would have plenty of opportunities to be together after the initial excitement of Margie's arrival home had settled.

The party was a huge success. Another real "Hurley bash." We were all running around in circles with the joy of having Margie home again, complete with her fiance and Master of Law degree. I was particularly happy and relieved to have my entire support group around me once again. We had all missed Margie so very much, especially Tarry.

Tarry arrived home from her holiday on July 28. She was sun-tanned (by sun and DDI), bright-eyed and appeared to be in very good health. She had even gained a little weight, was eating and sleeping well and seemed very relaxed and happy. No serious illness had presented for all of that year. Life was wonderful again for her.

Tarry was to enjoy the added bonus of a week in Surfers Paradise with us (an annual event). The day after we all came home, on Saturday, September 14, I took Tarry and her sisters to see Paco Pena and his flamenco dancers at the Victorian Playhouse at the Arts Center. Tarry was ecstatic. It was a marvelous, wildly Spanish concert which transported us all back to Spain for one exotic afternoon.

By now my massage practice was thriving. It was wonderful for me, but not so good for Frank. He was having great trouble keeping himself occupied. I felt almost guilty for being so successful. It was such happy work and so interesting and rewarding. For the most part, my clients and I had a great mutual rapport. I really looked forward to those two-and-a-half days work.

But what about Frank? Margaret and Stephen came to the rescue. The traveling companions who had joined us in the Cardinal Newman pilgrimage in England coaxed us into learning to play the game of bridge. This was a wonderful introduction to a whole new world of companionable activity. As time went by and life at home became more difficult, bridge became a vital player in the role of maintaining our sanity.

This card game requires the undivided attention of the players, and Frank showed great skill and interest as we attended the weekly lessons with our friends, with whom we still play once or twice a week. This has been a major contributing factor in the restoration of a normal routine in our lives since Caroline died. It was, and is, imperative to keep as occupied and active as possible. We were very fortunate to have such caring friends who could see our predicament and help us do something positive about it.

Frank also became more interested in playing golf, once again, thanks to the encouragement of his friends, with whom he really enjoys playing. We both find the stress of competitive golf unpleasant and exhausting, but the social, relaxed game is always good fun. In other words, we found it a good idea to try everything possible. Some things suited and others did not. But at least some activity was planned for nearly every day of the week.

Caroline's godmother, who is also one of my closest friends, arranged for me to accompany her to the series of Saturday afternoon symphony concerts at the Melbourne Concert Hall. This was wonderful for me. We could meet up early for a chat, and then lose ourselves in the wonder of the music for two whole hours. I always looked forward to these wonderful Saturday afternoons of peace and beauty with my dear friend, Jill.

She was like a fairy godmother to Caroline, and still is one to me. From day one of Caroline's illness, a life-belt had been thrown to the terrified mother and daughter as they floundered around in the dark waters of AIDS. Every time we tugged on that line for help, Jill would be there to support us so quietly and unobtrusively, with love, comfort and common sense, right up to, and beyond, the end of Caroline's life.

Carefully chosen books on eastern philosophies and astrology, two of Caroline's favorite topics for spiritual study, would arrive in the post along with a selection of tapes for relaxation and meditation. Caroline really loved and appreciated her wonderful godmother, who had been with me at school and at St Vincents. We have always shared the joys and sorrows of being wives and mothers. She is a very special person indeed.

More excitement was to come. On Saturday, September 28, Jamie and Sally announced their engagement. We were all so happy for them. Sally would be a very welcome addition to our family. She was already loved as a daughter and a sister by us all. The wedding was planned for April 3, 1992, just four weeks after Margie and Peter's wedding.

We were in for a very busy time. Once again, my heart missed a beat. Please God, keep Tarry well for this occasion too!

On Thursday, November 7, a package was delivered to our front door. It was small and square, and came from New York. In it were the DDC tablets we had ordered for Tarry. I took the parcel from the courier, signed for it and brought it inside and just stood and looked at it. I was really frightened. What if the DDC made her really sick or even killed her? No one could tell if the dosage of each tablet was too high or too low. It was such a terrible gamble, and Tarry had been so well for such a long time now.

I said nothing about their arrival for a few days. When I did tell her, she insisted on starting them immediately, with her doctor's permission, of course. The situation was one of all care but no responsibility, however. I felt physically ill as I watched Tarry swallow that first white and very large tablet. I really thought I would faint. I didn't, though, and managed to hide my fears behind a cup of tea. Tarry just swallowed the tablet, had a cup of tea as well, and showed no apprehension at all.

No apparent changes were to appear for a long time, so the opinion was that the tablets must be doing some good, or doing nothing. Tarry's state of health seemed to be remaining constant. This was a great blessing and would mean we could proceed with the wedding plans without worrying whether she could fully participate in this joyous event.

A beautiful suit was bought for Tarry, dark green with a very short skirt to show off those lovely legs, a white silk shirt edged in the same shade of green, matching Louis XIV heel shoes, and a pearl necklace and earrings to complete the outfit. She looked stunning. A very different rig-out from her usual uniform of blue jeans or leggings and multi-colored Mexican or Chinese tops.

Everyone had something new and special to wear. Dominique shone as the only bridesmaid to be dressed in white silk and Kristen looked lovely in her carefully chosen suit and hat. We were all highly excited and well organized. All the outfits were hung on padded hangers and stored away until the morning of March 7.

It seemed no time at all before Christmas Day was with us. It was so specially happy with all the family together again. This year the main topic of conversation revolved around the two weddings so close together. When the day was over, Tarry went back to Brunswick with her house mates and friends. They would celebrate New Year's Eve there together.

She visited us at Portsea from time to time over the next four weeks. Summer passed uneventfully. The weather was rather cold, so we spent the time writing out wedding lists and invitations and hoping warmer weather would herald in the autumn, to provide an Indian summer.

I resumed my massage practice, and the bridge and golf got under way again. Everything was proceeding like clockwork. We had been a normal family for nearly a whole year. I had actually become quite complacent about AIDS. Tarry was fine, or she seemed to be, and Frank was showing signs of becoming better adjusted to his retirement. The two weddings had raised his level of interest and happiness to a great degree. He was so delighted that Jamie and Sally were being married in the chapel of his, his father's and Jamie's old school. It was also to take place on the day that Frank's father would have celebrated his 100th birthday.

The source of his greatest joy was Tarry being so well and busy with her own life. We didn't know much about her activities, which I thought was a very good sign of independence regained and maintained. She checked in at least once a week and was always bright and chirpy. Monday nights were consistently reserved for the family roast beef (not even dinner with Tom Cruise would keep them away). They were wonderful nights, but have been abandoned now as one or other of the group has to work or is otherwise engaged. So we were lucky it worked while Tarry was still alive.

It was around this time that I received a notice from the Society of Clinical Masseurs Inc., of which I am a member. It contained particulars of a one-day workshop which would concentrate on the demonstration and practice of massage care of people with HIV/AIDS. It was to be held in a home in Brunswick one Saturday in May. I thought about this for a while and then decided to enrol.

It was an amazing and profoundly moving experience. I did not admit to any prior acquaintance with AIDS. Confidentiality was still a priority. All the patients were men, and one or two of them were very ill.

They stoically and generously submitted to being the focus of attention, while the hands-on demonstration massage was carried out. This, of course, was done by experts.

I watched the experienced masseurs lead the workshop with gentleness, compassion, concern and competence, and noted the warm, overwhelming empathy between them and the patients. As the day progressed, I knew in my heart that this was what I should be doing, too. I was already happily doing this for Tarry, as it was a wonderful way in which to comfort her while keeping a discreet eye on her physical condition.

I joined the roster of volunteer masseurs, and I am so glad that I did. One Saturday morning per month for nearly a year I had the privilege of providing therapeutic massage care for men with HIV/AIDS. It was wonderful to see each person respond with a feeling of warmth, well-being and relaxation. They each knew, for I had told them, that I was well acquainted with AIDS because of Tarry, and we had a special affinity, those patients and I. I really loved them all.

After the massage was completed, we would often have a chat over a cup of coffee. Their stories were all so sad and distressing and were deeply moving. Their pain and loneliness was quite palpable. I saw the really destructive and grassroots side of AIDS through their eyes. For the most part, they were all alone, with partners dead or gone away, and almost no family ties, if any at all. I will never forget those Saturday mornings and the people I met. It made me realize how fortunate Tarry was to have the support of family and friends to care for her and love her so unconditionally.

The patients always enquired after Tarry with genuine concern. They themselves were such generous and caring people. For me, it was an enriching and humbling experience. These young, and not so young, men did as much for me as I seemed to do for them. We would give each other a big hug and kiss goodbye and look forward to the next time.

That year was so special for me, I loved each visit so much, and eagerly anticipated those precious Saturdays. After Tarry died, however, I just couldn't go back again. I simply didn't have the physical or emotional strength to continue. I miss it, though, very much, and I do hope those special people are still alright. When I left the roster, none had developed full-blown AIDS.

CHAPTER 10

ॐ

THE TIDE TURNS

I awoke early on Saturday, March 7, 1992, got up and went downstairs to make a cup of tea and toast for Frank and myself, gathered up the morning paper from the driveway and went back upstairs with all this balanced on a tray. Just like any other Saturday? Not like any other Saturday at all! We sipped our tea and ate our Vegemite toast, leaving the papers unread while we anticipated the events of the coming day. I was quivering with excitement and nervous too, as I ticked off items on a long list of things to be done. For this was Margie and Peter's wedding day. And what a day it was. Warm, sunny and still. A perfect autumn morning. The four sisters assembled at Kew to get ready. Excited fingers (with beautifully manicured nails, for a change) produced much rustling of tissue paper and clacking of coat hangers as each of the outfits to be worn was laid out on the old familiar beds.

In the midst of all the flurry of hair-dos, make up, and 'baggsing' the bathroom, to which the girls were making frequent trips, I found myself suddenly overcome with feelings of apprehension. I couldn't understand it. It wasn't mother of the bride (awful phrase) jitters. Everything was proceeding so smoothly. Margie looked radiant in her bridal gown from Boston – all French lace and a long satin ribbon tied at her waist. The others looked beautiful, the flowers were gorgeous, and I had scrubbed up quite well in my special Italian suit. So what was wrong with me? Why was I feeling like this? Why today of all days?

The answer was standing straight in front of me. Tarry had been enthusing, almost hysterically, about what a wonderful day it was, how lovely everyone looked, how lucky Margie was and then suddenly she had stopped talking. She was unable to continue. Her chortly chattering just stopped dead. Luckily the others were very engrossed with what they were doing and didn't appear to notice any change in tempo. I looked at Tarry and I saw tears of real pain in her eyes.

I knew the cause of this pain. She would never be a bride herself, or more importantly, she would never be a mother. She had always longed for a child of her own and had actually discussed with me the pros and cons of AIDS and motherhood some time previously. After consulting various medical opinions, it had been considered that if Tarry should become pregnant, she would have to cease all medication for the unborn baby's safety, thereby hastening her own death. If her pregnancy went to term and the baby was delivered safely, it would surely have HIV, as Tarry was into the well-advanced stages of full-blown AIDS. This, in turn, would mean the eventual and certain death of her baby in addition to her own death. There was no way Tarry could endure all this: to have a baby and to die, and to have that baby die as well. I know Frank and I could never have survived so great a sorrow. It was an unthinkable situation. Tarry and I both knew this and we never discussed it again.

Of course Tarry knew that Margie was planning to start a family straight away, and now that the wedding was here, she felt sure that an announcement of a baby on the way would soon be made. I guess mixed in with the sadness was a small measure of jealousy, a very understandable feeling.

With the help of a small glass of champagne, which went straight to her head Tarry, managed to cheer up. She was jolly again. The cloud had passed. We both put on our powder and paint and joined the others for the photography session before leaving for the church. The photographer was a great enthusiast. He had everyone lined up left, right and center for photographs of groups inside the house and out in the garden.

One very special photo was taken of Frank and his four daughters under the golden poplar tree where Tarry had planted her daffodils two years previously. It turned out to be the most beautiful photograph of all. It stands in a special frame, on "Grandma's desk," always with a little crystal vase of flowers beside it. It was the last picture taken of Tarry and her sisters while she was still well.

Everyone joined together in enthusiastic celebration of this wonderful marriage of Margie and Peter. It was a magic day.

It also happened to be Newmarket Day, another important occasion for horse-racing fans in Melbourne. Frank and some of the guests had little transistors plugged into their ears to listen to the races during the afternoon. Someone took a photo of this group. They looked like a bunch of deaf old men allowed out for a special occasion. It all added to the fun and, in a happy way, poked a bit of fun at the extreme elegance of this day.

Frank had placed a bet on a filly named *Love Comes to Town* on his way from the church to the reception, and the horse won. When this news was included in Frank's proposal of health to the bride and groom, it brought the house down.

Four weeks later it was Jamie and Sally's wedding, on a clear, hot, Indian summer's evening. This was a really raucous occasion and overwhelmingly happy. The guests were nearly all young people ready to rock around the clock, and indeed they did.

Tarry had pushed aside her problems and looked really well and radiant as she danced the night away. It was fortunate for her, and for us, that we were unaware more trouble was on its way for her. No spanners would be thrown into her works, though, until a few days after the second wedding day.

Her next problem was thrush, or candidiasis, which is a fairly common (and in females, a very irritating) infection, and usually can be relieved by appropriate medication. Tarry had probably been suffering from a mild form of it for a while, but I only became aware of her situation when it began at this stage to affect her digestive tract. Because the AIDS virus weakens the natural immune systems so seriously, the usual remedies are much less effective. In Tarry's case, the infection was never entirely eliminated from her system for the rest of her life. It was to interfere intermittently with swallowing, digestion, and elimination. Her general well-being, and particularly her weight, were being progressively and adversely affected. Recurrent and frequent flare-ups of the infection over the next 12 to 14 months of her life resulted, quite understandably, in bouts of depression and irritability.

Tarry was still living at Brunswick, but seemed rather disenchanted with the boyfriend. She did not discuss this with me at all, but I later discovered that this was associated with his drug problems, which were by then getting out of hand. He was becoming less in control of his life, and more and more dependent on Tarry, who in turn was becoming less able to deal with all this stress.

She moved from Brunswick to live with Dominique in Parkville for a while. This would have been successful had she been left alone to look after her own needs, but she was being relentlessly pursued, either by phone calls or visits, at any time of the day or night, by this young man. It was becoming very hard for her to manage her life.

At this stage, there was nothing I could do. Tarry was adamant that she would not return to Kew unless she was really ill. As this was the original arrangement we had made, I had to stick with it. I found this extremely hard to deal with, but Dominique was very solicitous in her care of her sister. Tarry, I realize, did not want me to know about her friend's involvement with heroin. She was amazing how she could juggle her two lifestyles, both at such variance with each other.

On April 25, Tarry, her sisters and I all trooped off to the Neil Diamond concert at the Tennis Center in Melbourne. It was a huge success. Tarry was in her element as she jumped up to dance to the tune of *Sweet Caroline*, one of Neil Diamond's best known songs, which he delivered with great flair and style. I felt he was singing directly to Tarry. She looked so radiantly happy that night.

Margie and Peter would soon be leaving on a trip to Russia: traveling on the Trans-Siberian Railway to Moscow and beyond. Would the travel bug ever leave our family? I could see that Tarry was green with envy on both counts, but she enthused along with the rest of us at the family farewell dinner on Sunday, May 3.

This holiday was an amazing experience for Margie and Peter. They felt quite safe and happy until they reached Moscow, where Margie landed in hospital with a threatened miscarriage. The hospital attendants thought it would be a good idea to complete this process. Thank God they didn't. It was a great relief to have them safely home again on June 11.

Margie's pregnancy drew her even closer to Tarry. They shared everything. They decorated the nursery together and both shopped for baby clothes and other equipment. It was wonderful to see them in action. Tarry was now genuinely solicitous of Margie, delighting in her sister's good fortune. It was such a healthy and positive reaction. A whole new life was beginning for all of us, with this tiny new life forming inside our Margie.

The bassinet that my parents had for me when I was a baby was being refurbished for use for the 21st time. I had been the first baby to use it. My two brothers and one sister and all of our children had been in this bassinet as newborns, and now the third generation was about to take up residence. My mother would have been overjoyed, but she and my father had died some years previously.

I was really rather glad that they were not around to see these hazardous days of our lives. AIDS had been unknown to them and I very much doubt that they could have dealt with this trauma at close quarters. Mum would have given it her best shot though. Strangely enough, I often felt that she was with me and supporting me through these distressing times. So, it seemed, was her sister, my wonderful Auntie Vera, who had been a Loreto nun and had died in 1987, a year before our bomb was to drop. I know that Auntie Vera would have understood. There was no one quite like Auntie Vera. She was a most · compassionate, loving and unshockable lady. She and my mother were a wonderful duo.

The prospect of being grandparents was a source of great joy for Frank and me. It gave added impetus to Frank's enjoyment of life. He was still having retirement troubles, although he was doing his best with gardening, bridge, golf, reading and a little writing. He always looked so anxious, and it wasn't all due to Tarry's illness.

I thought I would help him along, by giving him a surprise birthday gift of a word processor, courtesy of my massage money. I had visions of him with this wonderful present, sitting at the dining room table all set and ready to type out a life of his beloved Cardinal Newman. On June 27, Frank's 72nd birthday, Tarry triumphantly carried in the wondrous word processor. Frank was surprised, but some years later, has still not mastered it. He keeps promising he will learn to use it, but I fear it will be obsolete by the time he gets around to it.

Tarry was spending more and more time at home with us at Kew. I think her main reason for living here was because it was warmer and a much more comfortable home than either Brunswick or Parkville. I was preparing all her meals, and intercepting unwanted phone calls from the ever-persistent boyfriend. I know she would have preferred to live independently, but there was really nowhere else where she could have lived so comfortably and securely.

Tarry was free to come and go as she wished, and most of the time she was an absolute delight to have around the house. She was mostly cheerful, although she had her ups and downs, which was accepted as normal, especially in the long, dark days of winter when often the bitter winds and driving rain belted the windows and rattled every door in the house. I sensed her loneliness of spirit, her longing for a normal, healthy life and love. Her need to give as well as to receive was intense and very obvious. I felt so frustrated and cross that she couldn't fulfill those needs to their fullest extent.

There were protected places in the garden where, on sunny days, Tarry would rug up and take her drawing pad and pencils and sit sketching for a while. Sometimes she would read. She read Lord of the Rings over again, as she did some works by Umberto Eco. But she looked pinched and anxious, as she had in her early days of AIDS, and she would soon lose interest in whatever she was doing, come inside again and lie down for a while looking very depressed.

These periods of depression became more and more protracted. She would curl up on the couch in the smoke room and just do nothing, or doze off. She looked so terribly ill during these times. Quite often she appeared to have just melted into the cushions and to be close to death. Although this was not the case, this was how she appeared to me, and it frightened me.

Tarry's psychologist, Donna, was very good to us both. Tarry would visit her frequently and always came home again after these visits in a much more buoyant mood. She was still practicing yoga and meditation each day, and when her energy levels were sufficiently high, she would walk down to the local municipal pool, which was heated and enclosed. There Tarry would dive in and swim many laps up and down, up and down with quite powerful and even strokes.

After she had walked home, I would massage Tarry for an hour. She really loved this and would usually then enjoy a reasonably substantial meal. After this she would sleep for at least two hours, and wake up refreshed and chirpy. If only those days could have lasted longer, for they were the very best days of all. We were so loving and close during those delicious days of peace. Still and all, I suppose we were fortunate to have them at all.

Tarry's "card girl" friends, ever loyal and loving, would call over and take her out to their homes, or to listen to a band at a bar. Tarry loved that. The "cardies" never allowed Tarry to feel left out, even when one by one they married and had their own babies. They shared all of this with their poor, sick pal, Caroline. The group never seemed to play any card game; it was all chatting, laughing and having fun.

This wonderful octet still keep in touch with me. They call in with their babies. They sent a beautiful potted rose to us for what would have been Tarry's 33rd birthday, and they have even invited me over for afternoon tea a – very thoughtful group. I love them all for loving Tarry as they did. It was this group that was to bring color and a touch of the old normal party atmosphere into Tarry's final days.

I kept the massage routine going with Tarry and it was with increasing alarm that I could see she was becoming thinner and thinner, despite all my efforts to keep her well nourished. It seemed to me as if it was the AIDS virus that was benefiting from all the nutriment in the food, leaving Tarry's vital organs to starve and waste away, too weak to fight for what was rightfully theirs. Three normal meals a day were becoming harder for Tarry to manage. The spirit was willing enough, but the flesh was just too weak. Small, frequent meals had now become the pattern, but even this routine was not very successful.

It was hard not to keep asking Tarry how she felt, whether she was taking her medication regularly, and also if she was remembering to keep her doctors' appointments. These things belonged in Tarry's province, and I knew if I interfered, it might drive her away from me. She did not want to discuss AIDS at all. But I could sense her increasing fear. Her face had become troubled and very lined. The texture of her skin was almost papery with dryness. This worried her, so I suggested to her that it could be the result of the almost constant exposure to our central heating. I gave her some special moisturizing cream to use, but it didn't seem to work very well. Once again, I made no comment. I was afraid she would resent me, as indeed she soon would, very bitterly, in the months to come.

Another physical problem had crept up on Tarry. She had developed peripheral neuritis of her legs and feet. This is a condition not unlike shingles, where the irritation of the nerve endings becomes almost unbearable with burning, itching pain. No rash or skin lesions were visible, apart from self-induced welts; the result of Caroline's desperate scratching in her search for relief. It was terrible for her, and upsetting to watch. Gentle, rhythmic massage, using a very light almond oil and stroking upwards from the feet, provided some respite and relief. I did this frequently, and Tarry would occasionally doze off on the massage table. The greatest source of relief, though, was vitamin B12. She had regular intramuscular injections of this at Fairfield with almost miraculous results.

Frank and I made the usual plans for our annual excursion to Surfers Paradise for three weeks in August. We decided to fly this time. We would have the first week on our own, then Margie and Tarry would join us for the second and third weeks.

The first and last weeks were a total disaster. On Sunday, August 9, Frank and I flew north, and there, for the first time in years, I was flattened by the flu. I was confined to bed for the whole of the first week of our holiday, and I was a miserable, resentful patient. The sun poured through the large window and sent daggers through my head; the light dancing off the ocean tortured my bloodshot eyes. I whined, slept, swallowed Panadol, mineral water and tea. How selfish I was to make such a fuss over such a minor complaint. I was in fact terrified of becoming really ill, and being unable to care for Tarry. I was also very afraid of passing on to her some germ that might prove fatal to her. My thinking was quite often distorted in this way.

By the time the girls arrived, all symptoms had gone, and we were all raring to go. The weather remained perfect and the four of us had a happy week together. Margie was in especially good form. She was very pregnant, and prettily so. She was revelling in the prospect of motherhood. We were constantly guessing as to whether a girl or boy would be born and tossing names around, sort of trying them out. It was really good fun but not for my Tarry.

Tarry, by contrast, looked even thinner than ever. Her tolerance and enthusiasm for the sun and sea had diminished. She had the occasional brief swim and then left the beach almost immediately she had dried off. In the old days, Tarry would be the first on to the beach, in and out of the surf like a dolphin, and the last to leave in the late afternoon.

It was so sad to see my true beach belle unable to enjoy her favorite pastime. One by one, all the lovely lights of Tarry's life were being extinguished, just as Margie was beginning to take hold of her exciting new world. I felt desperately torn between sorrow for one and joy for the other.

Sometimes in the afternoons Tarry would stroll into Cavill Avenue with Margie and me, but more often she would sleep or go for long, slow, solitary walks along the sand, heading away from Surfers Paradise, towards Southport. She sometimes found perfectly formed scallop shells, which she would give to me. We used to think they brought good luck. God knows why. I kept all those shells, and after Tarry died, I sprayed them silver and gold and arranged them on the Christmas table in a special basket. They will always be used at Christmas time.

We dined out on most of the evenings that Margie and Tarry were both with us at Surfers Paradise. Margie ate with a voracious appetite; feeding for two, of course. Tarry picked at her food, her mind far away. She was always restless and anxious to return to the flat. There were shadows deepening under her blue-green eyes, her cheeks were hollow-ing out and I was so afraid.

Margie returned to Melbourne after a week. She was missing her husband and was anxious to get home to him, all glowing and gorgeous as she was. Soon after she departed, Tarry was once more afflicted with the peripheral neuritis. She was absolutely and relentlessly tormented by the raging, invisible itch. She was in agony. I massaged her legs for hours on end. As soon as I stopped, the itching would return. We tried dipping her legs into buckets of iced water, and wrapping them in cold, wet towels to numb them. Her feet had "wires in them," so walking became sheer torture for her. We rang the doctor at Fairfield, who was out. She rang back, and we were out.

Then I remembered the vitamin B12. I went to a chemist, and it was like getting blood out of a stone. When the pharmacist was told the nature of the illness for which the injection was being used, he backed off and abruptly dismissed us. I was really upset and furious about this. To encounter a chemist like this on the Gold Coast, of all places; so many itinerant, intravenous drug users were continually passing through, no doubt acquiring syringes and needles as they went, possibly some of them with HIV, and yet when we had told the truth, we were turned away. We finally managed to get what we needed from another, more compassionate and understanding pharmacist. I was in tears at this stage, but at least I had the necessary help.

I administered the full course of injections to Tarry, but they had very little effect. She could barely sleep at night. She dozed on and off during the day and was too miserable to eat. She had cups of tea and orange juice, and the occasional Cornetto ice cream. She was irritable, and who could blame her? We eagerly awaited our flight to Melbourne on Saturday, August 30. Oh, what blessed relief it would be to be home again, and within reach of proper care for Tarry from her own doctors at Fairfield.

On our return Tarry went straight out to Fairfield, where after examination, her doctor immediately ceased the DDC. This drug of unknown dosage was what was causing all the trouble. After a very short time, the itching stopped completely and never returned.

Once Tarry had stopped taking the DDC, she began to feel much better. She was eating more, and she looked more relaxed. She asked me if I would go to Portsea with her on the following weekend, just the two of us. I was delighted to say yes.

We drove there on Friday afternoon. For dinner, which we had by the fire, we had fresh oysters (Tarry's favorite), fish and salad and a Cornetto each. These ice cream cones had become a ritual with us. We chatted and watched telly for a while, then went to bed early. Tarry slept like a log, but I didn't. I had a feeling we were at Portsea for some special reason of hers, and I was trying to work out what it could be.

Saturday was a beautiful day: warm and sunny without any wind. Tarry slept long and late, and seemed very well indeed when she emerged at midday, dressed and ready for a walk along the back beach. We took some sandwiches and orange juice in little cardboard packs, and we strolled along towards London Bridge, where we sat down to eat, feed the seagulls, and watch the waves booming under and around the immense rocky arch. The ferocious undertow, filled with trees of kelp, would suck the water, all hissing and boiling, back through the arch and out over the rocky ledge. These conditions were similar to those that in 1967 had claimed the life of Prime Minister Harold Holt at Cheviot Beach, just around the corner from where we were sitting. When the sea is like this, it is always an awesome sight, one that Tarry had loved from her childhood days. In previous times she used to climb to the top of London Bridge, but she no longer had sufficient strength.

As we sat looking out to sea, Tarry turned to me, and after some hesitation, asked if I would arrange for her to be cremated after she died, and then have her ashes scattered into the ocean from London Bridge.

I started shivering inside. So this was the reason for our pilgrimage to Portsea. I looked at her, put my arms around her thin little shoulders and said that of course I would arrange that for her. Then I hesitated before asking her if we could perhaps 'save' a little bit of her for a proper burial, just to keep the Catholic contingent happy.

Tarry managed a giggle and said that would be fine, but only if her grave could be in the Sorrento cemetery, facing west towards the ocean. Done, I said. We shook hands on this, gave each other a big hug, and walked back along the beach to the car and back to the fireside and cups of tea. I could feel the beginning of an oil slick of sadness seeping through and around my insides, a sensation which would never leave me completely. "Surely death is still a long way off," my heart said. "Perhaps not," my head replied.

After dinner that evening, Tarry hopped into bed beside me for a cuddle and a back rub. Then she asked me to say nothing of what had passed between us. I kept that promise. I really felt quite privileged that she had shown enough confidence in me to make such a request. I said nothing at all until the day she died, and Tarry never referred to that conversation again. She knew I would arrange things for her. She did not mention death for a long time after that day.

CHAPTER 11

჻

TURBULENT WATERS

On our return to Melbourne, I would notice more and more changes taking place in Tarry with each week that went by. These changes were to be irrevocable changes in her behavioral pattern, and swings in her mood. It seemed that her brain was becoming affected, either by the AIDS virus or the large quantities of medications she had been taking for nearly three years, or a combination of both. I was unaware at that time of any recreational drug use.

Tarry seemed to have patched things up with the boyfriend once again, and had moved back to Brunswick. I was really alarmed by this turn of events. It was such a sudden reversal of her recent patterns, but there was nothing I could do about it.

I kept myself busy with my massage practice and voiced my fears to no one, except Tarry's godmother, who comforted me as always. I had to be content with Tarry's arrival on odd occasions for a meal. She was usually accompanied by a large basket of washing to be done, hers and the boyfriend's. This was something new. She had always attended to her own laundry (when she was well, of course) but now it was just dumped by the washing machine as she proceeded on her way through the kitchen to plonk in front of the TV.

At first I was really annoyed by this, but then I realized that this, too, was part of the emergence of the very sick girl that Tarry was becoming in mind as well as body. So again I said nothing to her. I was sick with worry, though. I couldn't see where this was leading. Could this be treated, or was Tarry really going mad, as some AIDS patients do?

"Could someone please tell me just what is going on?" I would scream inside myself.

I was feeling really lonely and helpless at this time. Frank had his own ways of coping with the changes in Tarry, which may have helped him, but which I found a bit disconcerting and alienating. I didn't know what to do, so I drove down to Portsea by myself, to try to pull myself together and sort out the clutter in my mind. I had to make some decisions about how to best manage Caroline, myself, and our entire household.

I set about drawing up a list of positive things for me to do, and not do, in order to achieve and maintain some balance in my life and keep my mind clear and focused on what must be done and what must be avoided. I called this collection of good advice for myself "My Ten Commandments for My Survival," and generally speaking, they were successful. As things became worse on the home front, I would select one item from this list each morning and try to follow it through for that day. This list is still in my bedside drawer and I have occasion to refer to it from time to time.

The list included the following:
- Do remember the good things about Caroline. Her bravery and courage in the face of disaster, the kindness she had always shown to me when she was well.
- Try to clear my mind of all the negative, hurtful and horrible aspects of Caroline's present behavior. It is entirely due to AIDS at work.
- Do not feel a failure with regard to Caroline. I have really tried everything to help her. I cannot prevent her death.
- Try to keep life in its true perspective, accept that Caroline will die, but don't anticipate when and how this will happen.
- Stop trying to ease Frank's retirement pain. It is his own responsibility to deal with this. It is not my fault that he is unhappy.
- Do not try to protect family and friends from Caroline; they must cope with her in their own way.
- Do not say "yes" when I mean "no" and do not apologize for things not done or forgotten.
- Try to keep up activities that I enjoy: play bridge, massage clients, get hair done once every week, go to the movies,. alone if necessary. Go shopping, but don't overdo this. Plan little holidays, even if I can't go away.

• Try to keep up appearances for my sake, not others, and confide
in no-one, except for the psychiatrist and Jill.
• Take time to enjoy the anticipation of Margie's baby. Enthuse
along with Margie and knit some more baby jumpers!

Writing down these ideas made me feel much better. The list is
exactly as I wrote it down at the time, and I am so glad I did this.
It did become rather hard to adhere to some of these rather idealistic
guidelines, though. Hopefully, it may be of some help to others in a
similar situation.

After a weekend of all this pondering, I returned to Melbourne, feeling refreshed and much better able to cope. Tarry seemed quite normal
again for a while. Her enthusiasm for the arrival of Margie's baby was
rekindled. She and I went over to Margie's place and admired the nursery
all over again. We helped Margie pack her case for hospital. Then Tarry
put away all the baby clothes in neat piles in the little white chest of
drawers, having first lined each drawer with lightly perfumed paper.

We took photos of each other standing beside the empty bassinet,
which was in readiness for its tiny new occupant, then the three of us
walked to the Royal Botanical Gardens, which were close by. We fed the
swans, admired the beautiful trees and flowers, especially the enormous
rhododendrons, which were in full and magnificent bloom. The "pink pearl"
was our favorite of the rhododendron bushes.

We also had a giggle at the courting couples dotted around the lawns
on that warm, sleepy spring afternoon. "Watch out!" Tarry would whis-
per. "You too could be in trouble!" What awful black humor.

On September 27, 1992, we all visited Jamie and Sally in their new
home for afternoon tea, and during our visit they made their own big
announcement. They too were expecting their first baby, some time late
in February 1993. Tarry was already with them when the rest of the
family arrived as Jamie and Sally had shown her the great kindness and
courtesy of telling her their news first. She was indeed happy for them,
but I could see her becoming quieter and sadder as the retelling of their
happy news to us brought out the cheers and champagne. For Tarry, it
also brought the tears to her eyes.

My heart bled for her. She would never have any good news of her
own to share. She looked so fatigued. Her cheekbones, more prominent

than ever, cast hollow shadows where once her plump and rosy cheeks had bloomed. Her hair was all dull and thin and wispy, and her shoulders were stooped and frail.

Tarry started doing strange and unusual things again. She began to call on Kristen, then Dominique, Jamie and Sally, and Margie and Peter. Unannounced and at any time of the day or night she would drive over and wander in. Then she would sit down to chat, or turn on the telly. She would carefully examine their books, records or compact disc collections, select what she fancied and claim these goods as her own. She would join them for a meal, or just have a cup of tea, then leave in her little green Corolla car as suddenly as she had arrived. Or then again, she might curl up on a couch and drop off to sleep.

Although I remembered the resolutions I had made regarding the rest of the family and Tarry, I had to say something. I told each of them how worried I was about Tarry upsetting and disrupting their households. I was also afraid they would resent her, and I knew I was powerless to prevent what she was doing.

They all reassured me that they were not at all inconvenienced by Tarry's comings and goings. They loved having her with them, they said, and in spite of her strange behavior, they felt very comfortable with her. They insisted that I must not worry and that I was not responsible for her actions. I was very grateful to them for adopting that attitude. They were so kind and loving towards their obviously very sick sister.

My full attention then turned to Margie, for her baby was due to arrive on or around October 30. Peace reigned again for a little while, a very little while indeed.

On the morning of Saturday, October 17, Frank and I were out doing some early shopping. We arrived home to find Peter and Margie's car in the drive. We ran inside thinking that Margie must have gone into early labor and they were on their way to hospital. We were quite wrong, however.

Tarry had arrived at Kew while we were out. There was no one at home. She had driven her car over from Brunswick all alone. Having discovered our absence, she had rung Margie and Peter asking them to come quickly. She was desperately ill and was terrified.

Margie and Peter raced over from South Yarra to find Tarry lying down on the couch in the smoke room with the curtains drawn. She had a raging headache, stiff neck, back pain, high temperature and photo-phobia, hence the darkened room. She was showing all the signs of having meningitis. The symptoms had struck suddenly in the early hours of the morning.

True to her promise, Tarry had come over to Kew. She hadn't thought of ringing before she left Brunswick; she just headed for her car and Kew. I was horrified to think she had driven on her own, so very ill, and in the stream of early morning traffic.

Peter had rung Fairfield, where a bed was waiting for Tarry in her old haunt, Ward Five. Margie had checked the contents of the ever-ready hospital overnight bag, adding a few little extras, including Tarry's faithful old teddy bear and the pink slippers. Frank and I helped Tarry into the car and laid her across the back seat on pillows. She wore sunglasses to protect her eyes from the painful light. We were convinced that she had contracted yet another AIDS-related condition, cryptococcal meningitis, which was a very dangerous and life-threatening illness

As soon as Tarry was settled into her bed, she was given a pain-relieving injection, which helped her very much. She was in a terrible state. She didn't want me near her as I bent over to stroke her forehead. Exhausted, she fell asleep, and we went home for a while.

Many tests were done on Tarry, including a lumbar puncture, but nothing abnormal was detected. It was the cruel, teasing AIDS virus assuming a new mantle for a few days in order to frighten Tarry and all of us. Indeed, by Monday, October 19 (my birthday again), Tarry seemed very much better, although she had to remain in hospital for a few more days.

After her discharge from Fairfield, Tarry stayed at home for two days, then insisted on returning to Brunswick. Once back in Brunswick, the random house calls to her family and friends resumed, but still noone seemed to mind. She continued to keep up her visits to her Chinese doctor, in whom she had great faith. He was always so good to her. It was a comfort to me to know he was keeping an eye on her, as well as treating her with acupuncture, special herbs, and "moxi-bustion," which is a type of old-fashioned "cupping," to release the toxins from her body, especially around her chest and back. She was having continuous problems with a hacking cough, which could have been residual from the pneumonia and tuberculosis.

About a week after Tarry's discharge from Fairfield, the wonderful news of the safe arrival of Greta Jane Hurley Mitchell was announced. Poor Margie had endured a long, protracted labor, culminating in a Caesarean section. Greta was born on October 30 (Derby eve). I couldn't believe that all these major happenings, good or bad, were always coinciding with important race days. This event brought perfect joy for us all. We were all beside ourselves. I think I called every relative and friend we had, and they all enthused with us. It was marvelous.

After we had visited Margie and her little Greta on Cup Day, Jamie and Sally, Kristen and Tarry came to keep me company at Kew. A most unusual thing had happened. It had absolutely poured with rain on Derby Day, and was pouring again on Cup Day. So much rain had fallen that the picnic areas of the car park were under water and, for the most part, were unusable and closed. Frank went out to Flemington, regardless, all waterproofed from head to toe. Nothing could dampen his enthusiasm for these special race days.

We spread out the picnic fare on the large square coffee table in front of the telly in the smoke room. We each wore one of my race hats. Jamie wore a peaked airforce cap that had belonged to his late Uncle John, better known as "Spot Hurley," Tarry's godfather. It was all a bit silly and we laughed a lot. Tarry joined in and had fun. She even backed Sub Zero, the winner of the Melbourne Cup that year.

Margie and little Greta came home from hospital on the following Saturday. She was still rather tired and shaky, but she had many willing helpers, including Tarry, who at first could not do enough to help Margie get into a routine with Greta. All her old organizing skills emerged. We were all delighted with the way she so capably handled this brand new domestic scene.

Her interest soon waned, though, and once more she took to her ramblings. Her behavior was becoming more and more erratic, and she would appear and then disappear. She was pilfering from friends and family, and accusing others, mainly me, of tampering with or stealing her belongings. This time I was really very alarmed.

I rang Tarry's psychologist, who agreed to see her at once. I also rang her doctor. She wanted to see her immediately, to have her neurologically assessed and, if necessary, given appropriate medication. The trouble was that while I was making these arrangements, Tarry had driven off again, and I had no idea where she had gone.

She had headed off to stay with friends at Wye River, about two hours southwest of Melbourne along the Great Ocean Road. They had been expecting her, and rang to tell me she had arrived safely but was very agitated. They said they would watch over her for the weekend and see her home safely on Monday. They truly were, and are, the most wonderful young people. The "card girls" were the nucleus of this group of friends. They showed no fear or distaste or criticism of their pal Tarry and AIDS. They loved her, warts and all, and did all they could to keep her comfortable and happy, whereas I could hardly hide my anxiety.

I had reached the stage where I had begun to think that there must be something I was doing or not doing that was aggravating Tarry's state of aggression, anger and haphazard wanderings. I knew, though, that Tarry had an appointment to see her doctor the following Monday, November 16, so I put my worry on hold for that weekend.

One of my main concerns at that time was Tarry's unheralded housecalls to Jamie and Sally. Sally had been feeling very unwell and needed lots of rest during the day to make up for her uncomfortable and largely sleepless nights. She was about five months into her pregnancy. Jamie had to work overnight at the hospital on occasions, leaving Sally on her own. Admittedly, she usually had a friend or family member to keep her company, but I felt that a sudden, unexpected nighttime visit from Tarry could frighten and upset her. I was really terribly worried about this.

I rang Jamie, whereupon he gently and quietly told me exactly what was happening to Tarry. These are his words to me, as I remember them. He said, "Mum, there is nothing you can do about this. Mum, darling Mum, you have to face the fact now that Caroline is dying. She is really dying. You have been and you are a wonderful mother. You have done everything possible for Tarry. You can't stop her erratic activities. Sally and I don't mind her calling over. It's our responsibility, not yours. You must stop taking everything on yourself. You have got to take care of yourself. We will look after ourselves and you, and between us all we will take care of Tarry. Please stop worrying so much. We'll adjust to what Tarry is doing."

I will never ever forget Jamie for that. It was so wonderfully kind of him to tell me this. At the same time it must also have been enormously difficult for him. If all his patients are as lucky as I was then, to be on the receiving end of such thoughtfulness and wisdom, then they are indeed very fortunate to be in his care.

I was in floods of tears by the time I had hung up the phone. I sat down with a cup of tea to absorb and digest the fact that we were now reaching the point of no return. Caroline was not just going to die one day, she was actually in the process of dying, perhaps within six months.

I was glad I was able to draw comfort from the teapot and not the brandy bottle, because in order to maintain as much peace and harmony as possible, I would need to be very clear-headed and careful in the way I handled Caroline, myself and others close to me from here on. Actually, I did fly off the handle on some occasions during the desperate days ahead. I couldn't help this. As some people might say, "The way to hell is paved with good intentions." My intentions were good, but I was already in hell, along with everyone else close to Caroline. Hell on earth, I mean.

In late November I rang a friend of Tarry who was associated with the Ian Gawler Foundation. I thought he might have some ideas to help Tarry. He suggested that a health resort that had been established near Coolangatta might be very beneficial for Tarry's physical and mental well-being; and at the same time I would get a break, knowing that she would be well looked after. Before I said anything to Tarry, I rang the resort to make sure that they were happy to have people with AIDS stay there, and that there would be no isolation or prejudice. I was reassured that Tarry would be most welcome.

I then told Tarry. She was delighted at the prospect of one more holiday in the warmth of Queensland, where she would be with people with whom she could relate. She fell about with thanks. The requested deposit was posted off for the week's stay, and a discount airline ticket purchased for Saturday, December 12, returning on the following Saturday in time for Christmas.

This time Tarry needed help with the packing, but no matter, she was so anxious to get there she did not care what she took with her. The pills were packed as usual, but they were not given much attention during this holiday. Ahead of Tarry lay a week of meditation, yoga, massage and a carefully (I hoped) worked-out diet that might boost her weight a little. All this combined with a routine of gentle exercise and congenial company had our Tarry on fire with excitement. I was so happy for her; we all were. Frank drove her out to the airport, while I stayed at home to prepare for Greta's christening party, which was being held here at Kew on the following afternoon.

Tarry really hated big gatherings now, so she was pleased she wouldn't be at this party. These gatherings embarrassed and confused her. She felt very uncomfortable with some people, as they did with her. Decorating the Christmas tree had been her contribution, and it was indeed a great help to me. I was equally as pleased as she was that she would not be here, for it meant that I could relax and focus my attention on Margie and Peter, and their newly christened "Greta the Gorgeous," as she was and is known. Kristen was chosen to be Greta's godmother and was so thrilled to be honored in this special way.

The whole occasion was very successful and lots of fun. Everyone made a great fuss of Greta, who smiled or slept through it all. All who enquired after Tarry were delighted to hear that she was enjoying the sun, the rest, and all the good things of the health resort.

Two days before Tarry was due to return home, we had a phone call asking if she could stay until Christmas Eve. She was having such a wonderful time, she said, and one of the guests was able to change her return flight to arrive at 2:30 pm in Melbourne on December 24. Of course we agreed to this, delighted that it was all working out so well.

With the knowledge that Tarry was safe and having such a good time, I was really free to put my heart and soul into Christmas. The Christmas shopping was done in a flurry of excitement in one day flat. There was something special for everyone and a little Christmas stocking with a little sparkly star on a wooden stick for Greta.

I attended a number of pre-Christmas lunch parties, all of which were great fun. I felt so happy with the world, because it seemed that Tarry was not as sick as we thought. Perhaps she would be with us for much longer than anticipated. I was really over the moon about this and so was Frank. The spirit of Christmas was everywhere.

Maria made the puddings again that year. She and all her family were coming for Christmas lunch. I had great fun decorating the dining room table, set for 16 guests. It looked lovely – silver and gold pine cones and candles on a red tablecloth with dark green table napkins. Alternating red and green bonbons were placed at each place setting. With tiny electric bud lights threaded through the indoor pot plants, it all looked like fairyland.

All I needed now was to see Tarry walk through the door on Christmas Eve looking refreshed, glowing and gorgeous once again, and my joy would be complete. On Christmas Eve, Frank triumphantly met Tarry at the airport to drive her home. But she didn't want to come to Kew. Instead she wanted to stay at Brunswick overnight and come home to us on Christmas morning.

I was bitterly disappointed when Frank came home without her. Frank said that she looked very well, and was full of enthusiasm about her holiday, but somehow I sensed that I was not getting the full story. Frank didn't enlarge on this. Together we completed the food preparations. Cold buffet was this year's menu, with hot Christmas pudding, of course.

We had a meal, just the two of us, after which we filled the children's Father Christmas stockings. This was a tradition we had kept up from the time they were born, and now, seeing that they were all around their early thirties, it had become quite a joke. All these great big adults would be rummaging around to find a packet of Smarties, underpants, socks, next year's diary, suncream, and various freebie samples of expensive face creams and lotions. The previous year Father Christmas had given Sally a small sample tube of anti-cellulite cream and anti-aging eye-wrinkle creme. She nearly killed me.

This was always great for a laugh, but Frank and I decided that this would be the last year for the stockings. We both knew, in our hearts, that Tarry would not be with us for Christmas 1993, so in future, the stockings would be for grandchildren only.

Tarry arrived at Kew around 11:45 on Christmas morning. Frank and I had just arrived home from Mass. I still couldn't go to Sunday Mass, but Christmas was different. Tarry did look well, in a way. She was very tanned and her eyes were lustrous and clear, but something was wrong. She was almost hyperactive at one instant, then suddenly she would sit down in silence. Then up she would jump again to let us know how much weight she had gained, which she hadn't. If anything, she was even thinner than before. She kept telling us over and over how much the people up there "loved" her. "They really loved me," she said.

I stated that would have been easy for them, as she was a very lovable person, adding that we loved her very much too, always had done and always would. She looked a bit uncertain after I said that and replied that was nice, but she would prefer to be with her new friends.

I couldn't believe my ears, and could barely contain the tears. That remark had really hurt. The next thing, Tarry was demanding a massage, there and then. The rest of the entourage were due to arrive in half an hour. However, I agreed to do this for her.

"Just my back, shoulders and head." No "please," no "thank you."

I seethed with rage.

"At your service, madam," I snarled inwardly, as I went to work.

She was indeed, alarmingly thin. I had to be careful not to massage her too deeply. Little by little, the wasting process peculiar to some, perhaps most, AIDS patients was making progress in Tarry. I felt ashamed for thinking those nasty, sarcastic thoughts about her. Fear at work in the two of us again.

That fear was escalating within Tarry and me, making us even more irritable and unreasonable with each other. It seemed to me as though Tarry was in the center of a circle, the diameter of which was gradually diminishing. The area left around her was filling up with the detritus of AIDS, and impending death was pushing us further apart. Tarry was retreating into a womb of solitary existence and I was having trouble keeping the umbilical cord patent and operating to provide any physical and emotional nourishment. Everything was working in reverse and it was a nightmare.

I was saved for the moment by the front door bell. Our guests had arrived en masse. I left Tarry covered up and almost asleep on the massage table in the smoke room, while I went into "Happy Christmas" mode. Soon after, Tarry emerged all animated once again to mingle happily with family and friends. I noted, with interest, the non-arrival of the boyfriend. I removed his place setting from the table and nothing was said.

Sally and Jamie were also unable to be with us. Jamie had been called into work, and Sally was in the maternity outpatients with stomach pains that might have been early contractions. She had to be in hospital all day for observation. So that year they had a rotten Christmas.

The rest of us had a jolly time, as we usually did at Christmas. Greta the Gorgeous, now nearly two months old, was the center of attention. She was so happy, content and very, very pretty. She still is. Everyone wanted to cuddle her.

My glance kept returning to Tarry with increasing sadness. It was so painful to watch her deep in animated conversation with those around her. She left the table as soon as she could and went upstairs, where a short time later I discovered her asleep, curled up on her bed and looking awful. She had tried with great spirit to help clear the table, something she had always tackled with efficiency, like greased lightning really, but this time it exhausted her. Quite often one or more of our guests would have a rest after the hearty Christmas meal, so no one took much notice of Tarry's departure from the dining room. She had eaten virtually nothing. She had ignored me for most of the day, and I was so wretchedly miserable I had a hard time hiding my feelings.

Luckily, we have some real comics in our family circle, especially Maria and Dominique's boyfriend. They had everyone in hysterics with their antics, so with their performances, and Greta's gorgeousness, I was mercifully spared from stacking on too false an act. Everyone did a sterling job of keeping the Christmas spirit on the boil, while I sat quietly on the back-burner for a change.

After everyone had left, Tarry decided to drive home to Brunswick. I packed up a good supply of leftovers for her to share with the other members of that household, hoping that Tarry would feel hungry enough to eat something herself.

Frank and I were going to Adelaide on New Year's Eve to attend the wedding of the youngest son of great friends of ours. Tarry spent most of that week between Christmas and New Year with us, and during that time she thawed out a bit towards me and told me more about her time at the health resort. She showed me a number of tins of different powdered substances, which when mixed with water and drunk were guaranteed to boost her immune system. What rubbish, I thought, and worse still, they were quite expensive and had not been paid for. I wrote out another cheque and gave it to Tarry to post.

During the course of another conversation, she came to light with something that really started my alarm bells ringing. She told me that there was a doctor there at the resort, a pathologist, who had examined her blood and had told Tarry that her white blood cells were the "wrong shape," and that that was why she had AIDS. If she took the prescribed powders on a regular basis, her blood cells would return to their "right shape" and the virus would leave her. I felt sure she was making this up, but rather than upset her by saying so, Frank and I just said that that was good to hear and let's hope it works, and left it at that. We hoped she might eventually lose faith in that idea.

Tarry then asked me for more money. She was broke, she said. I gave her another cheque. She asked me not to tell her father and that she would repay me when she could. I did not know then that this money was being used to support the boyfriend's heroin habit. Her life was so miserable with him, but she said nothing. She was drawing further away from me.

One day, during that same week, I was outside lying by the pool. I looked up to see Tarry sitting upright and fully clothed on a sun lounge in the shade under the jacaranda tree. She was staring at me from behind little round dark John Lennon sunglasses, with an expression of sheer hatred.

I got up, went into the kitchen and burst into tears. What had I done wrong this time? Then the penny dropped: I was middle aged, healthy and alive and my daughter was young, diseased and dying – slowly dying of AIDS – and this was making her hate me (perhaps *resent* might be a better word to use).

This resentment was to continue for most of the next five months. It is not unusual for carers of very ill people to be given a hard time, especially when the illness is AIDS. These patients are usually quite young people who have lived adventurous and independent lives and they are bitterly resentful of their illness and certain death. Their feelings of anger and frustration explode around their closest carers, who in Tarry's case was me. It was desperately hard to take. We had been such pals, she and I, all her life, and through her illness up until now. I knew this was all part of the process, but it really didn't make things easier. I pulled my "Ten Commandments" out of the bedside drawer for another look and a touch of reassurance. They did at least help a little.

Frank and I flew off to the wedding in Adelaide on New Year's Eve. It was wonderful. We had such a happy time with our close and caring friends. It was the last happy gathering we would be part of for a very long time. As we all held hands to sing *auld lang syne* at midnight, I prayed that "auld acquaintance would not be forgot" as we peered into the darkness of 1993.

We arrived home in Melbourne on Saturday, January 2, and immediately packed the car and drove to Portsea. I had noticed an advertisement in that Saturday's paper for a weekend away for people who were very ill but still able to get around. It would be a weekend of massage and meditation, and included an introduction to the techniques of massage whereby one sick person would be shown how to massage another sick person.

This seemed like a great idea to me, and when I told Tarry, it did to her also. In fact she leapt at the prospect of mixing with new people who were also ill, and the idea of trying her hand at massage appealed to her very much. Sometimes, when things are really going wrong, bad feelings can be improved by doing something nice for someone else. Tarry and I both subscribed to that theory.

During most of the two weeks that Frank and I were at Portsea, Tarry was in Melbourne. She had started to give away a number of her possessions to special friends. She had a large poster of the Sistine Chapel Ceiling which we had bought together in Rome in 1983. This was framed and hung on the family room wall, for me, and it is still there. She was also spending time browsing around secondhand bookshops in search of suitable books for Greta and the babies of her friends. She inscribed all of these quite beautiful and well-chosen children's books with the same quotation:

> *To see the world in a grain of sand*
> *And Heaven in a flower*
> *Hold Infinity in the Palm of your hand*
> *And Eternity in an hour.*

"AGE OF INNOCENCE"
WILLIAM BLAKE

I suspected at this time that doctors' appointments and tablet-taking were being ignored or forgotten. To be fair to Tarry, she was not think-ing at all clearly. Her mind and memory were deteriorating, and I could see that she was becoming more bewildered and frightened. She did not mention this at all. I knew, also, that she was pinning her hopes on her blood cells resuming their "right shape." All we could do for now was just be there for her, and not ask questions, which would surely antagonize or confuse her.

As well as giving her things away, Tarry was becoming morbidly suspicious of other people. She felt they were cheating her in some way. Her bankbook was "stolen;" it was in the zip-up section of her shoulder bag. Somebody had "stolen" her favorite (at that time) CD, "My Friend the Chocolate Cake;" I replaced it, and then replaced it a second time. I finished up with three copies of this New Zealand group's music. Luckily I liked their music very much, especially their rendition of *Danny Boy* or the *Londonderry Air*.

In other words, nothing had been stolen, but everyone came under suspicion for something or other. Even the CD player I had given Tarry for her birthday in 1991, she found to be faulty. It wasn't. But I had the finger pointed at me for delivering damaged goods to her doorstep. She threw it back at me and that was the end of that. It was all so desperately out of character, so heartbreakingly sad.

On Friday, January 15, off Tarry drove to Yarra Junction, a bit over an hour's drive east of Melbourne, for her weekend of meditation.

She had seen her doctor and promised faithfully to see her again after she returned from this weekend's activities. On that same day, Frank and I bought Tarry a new bed for her room at Portsea. She had been complaining for some time that the bed springs were all sagging, which left her with a constant backache. She was right about the bed, and we were glad to replace it for her. Her backache was also caused by a strange thickening and swelling in her lower right lumbar region, just above her now very prominent pelvic bones. I had noticed this lump and it was quite firm during one of our massage sessions. I never found out what the diagnosis was. Everything seemed to be happening so quickly.

After her weekend away, Tarry arrived at Portsea on Monday, January 18, saying that she really had not enjoyed her time there very much at all. The other people were so ill, she said, and she was the only well person in the group. Then she disappeared suddenly, without saying where she was going. Dominique rang to say that Tarry had caught the ferry from Portsea across the heads to Queenscliff and was with her at Dominique's boyfriend's family beach house at nearby Point Lonsdale.

Her arrival had not been an unannounced one. They had received a phone call from Tarry asking to be met at the ferry. She had forgotten to tell us she had arranged to do this. Well, at least we knew where she was, and she was going to stay overnight at Point Lonsdale with her sister and friends. She would return to Portsea the following morning.

This suited us very well, for we had been invited to Red Hill on Westernport Bay to play golf and stay overnight with friends from Sydney. The wife was an old friend of mine from school and nursing days. We had not seen this couple for some time, and this was an excellent opportunity to catch up. Or so I thought.

Unfortunately I was so wrapped up in Tarry's present condition that I kept losing the thread of the conversation. Naturally enough, these kind friends were anxious to know how Tarry was faring and I was becoming more and more agitated as I answered their questions. It was no one's fault. I knew something was really, really wrong and I just had to get back to Portsea. We left soon after breakfast, and drove straight back along the freeway. I was exhausted. I had not slept at all that night.

As we turned into the drive and got out of the car, Tarry came flying down the back steps from the kitchen, screeching on top note at us: "I'm cured! I'm cured! The virus has gone! I no longer have AIDS! I'm going to live forever! You must be so happy for me!"

We stood rooted to the spot. I was frozen with shock. Tarry ceased her tirade, looked at us and said, "You don't believe me, do you? You don't believe me! You don't believe that I'm cured! Why don't you believe me?" and she burst into tears, all pale and trembly.

Frank just said quietly, "How do you know you are cured, darling? What happened while we were gone?"

Tarry then told us how she had recently taken some blood by pricking her fingertip, had placed it on one of Frank's old pathology glass slides, and posted it up to the Queensland pathologist, who had just rung her at Portsea to tell her the wonderful news that her blood cells were now in their normal shape; she was cured of AIDS.

This was real nightmare territory. What on earth were we going to do now? Poor Tarry really thought we would believe this fabricated tale of quackery, a tale she so desperately wanted to believe herself. Poor darling girl, it hadn't worked out the way she hoped.

She was absolutely furious with us. She disappeared back inside, but before long had reappeared. She flew into her car, leaving her pills and belongings behind. Without looking left or right or behind, she reversed out of the drive nonstop into Blair Road and set off at a screaming pace for Melbourne. Where in Melbourne she was going we had no idea, nor whether she would arrive there safe and accident-free. We didn't know what to do.

We went back into the house and made ourselves a hot, comforting pot of tea to give ourselves time to calm down. There was no point in following her. This would surely cause an accident. Before deciding on any action, it seemed better to wait for at least an hour and a half, which under normal driving conditions is the time it takes to reach Melbourne from Portsea.

While we waited, I rang Fairfield and told the girl on the switchboard what had happened and asked her to contact the doctor and the man at the hospital security gate so that if Tarry did go there, her arrival could be reported back to us. But Tarry did not turn up at

Fairfield. I rang various friends of hers, and my sister. No one was expecting her, but they would let us know if she turned up within the next two hours. We were both desperately worried and frightened for Tarry's safety.

I went into her little Portsea room, which looked over the garden facing west, the aspect Tarry loved so much, and it was my turn for tears. Her room was in chaos. Anything mobile had been hurled around the room in her rage. Pills were everywhere – under the bed, in corners, under pillows, mixed up with spilt coffee and squished cigarettes, half-smoked. Scarves, socks and half-eaten sandwiches were lying every-where among the bedclothes that had been tossed around the room. It was a terrible sight, and it broke my heart. Worse was to come, however.

After two hours without hearing any news, we locked up the house and drove home to Kew. I knew that Tarry had an appointment with her doctor late that morning. I had made a note of it in my diary. I therefore felt reasonably sure that she would eventually arrive at Fairfield. Meanwhile, it seemed that our best option was to go straight home and await any news there.

When we arrived home, Tarry's car was in the driveway. We rushed into the house and found Tarry in the smoke room. A completely strange Tarry; surely this couldn't be our Tarry. But it was. This stranger was sitting cross-legged on the floor. She had just-dyed, wispy black hair, and the dye was dripping through the towel around her shoulders and onto the carpet. She was rocking back and forth, back and forth, humming a little ditty to herself. There was the strange high-pitched screechy sound of an Indian sitar coming from the record player.

She was surrounded by scraps of brightly colored fabric, which she was trying to sew together. She looked up at me, and I hardly recog-nized her. She said: "Now that I am cured, I'm going to make a dress for myself and Maria is going to show me how to do it. Look at this beautiful material, this will be my special new dress. I am so happy. I am so happy." She kept rocking, and her voice faltered and faded as she repeated these words over and over. I knew the time had come to take a stand. Frank couldn't, he was too upset. But I could. I had to. She simply had to go to hospital, and right now.

My heart was racing all over my chest. Quite loudly and evenly I said to Tarry, "You had an appointment with the doctor this morning, and you didn't keep it."

"How do you know?" asked Tarry.

"Because I rang Fairfield. You just disappeared from Portsea this morning. Dad and I were terribly worried about you. You are coming to Fairfield with me right now."

"I will not, you bitch! I'm cured!" Tarry yelled right back at me. It was awful for Frank caught between the crossfire of this slanging match between his wife and daughter.

"You can say what you like, darling," I said, "but you are coming with me, to Fairfield, right this very instant."

I had her overnight bag, which was always at the ready, in one hand and I held Tarry's hand with the other, to lead her to the car. Frank rang Fairfield and we were told to take Tarry straight to outpatients. The doctor would be waiting for us there. Tarry, furious, belligerent and stony-faced, sat bolt upright in the back seat of the car. Dye was still seeping from her hair down the back of her flimsy Indian cotton dress, which was see-through. This made Tarry look infinitely worse, particularly as she was not wearing her undies. I hadn't noticed this before we left home, but I thought I would be able to tie a scarf across her hips when we arrived.

Tarry wouldn't let me touch her, and she was too sick and angry to care about what she was, or was not, wearing. She stormed ahead of us along the corridor to OP. She would have nothing to do with me at all. She kept running ahead, while I tried to catch up. I felt weepy and wrung out by this stage. The bravado was deserting me, and my hated oil slick of sadness was once again slipping over and around my insides. I felt sick and faint with anxiety.

Tarry stomped into the OP department and announced her arrival to the receptionist. She stormed around to the doctor's office, where of course, she had to wait. She couldn't just barge in there. Frank and I stood aside and let her go. We had no idea what to do.

The doctor emerged from her consulting room looking very concerned. She told Tarry that she would have to be admitted for a while to be carefully examined. Poor Tarry now realized that no one was going to believe her story about her miraculous cure.

I stepped forward to go with Tarry up to the ward – Ward Four this time, not her usual Ward Five – and she pushed me away. She lunged towards me again, and pushed me once more. She grabbed the overnight bag from me and almost ran off to Ward Four with the nurse who had come to admit her. People were staring, open-mouthed, at us. They had obviously not seen a girl with this condition before. I burst into tears on the doctor's shoulder. She did her best to comfort me, saying all the while what a terrible disease AIDS is.

It certainly is. It had destroyed my beautiful daughter – eating away at her, and turning her into a scrawny, screeching bundle of terror and misery. I couldn't stand seeing her like this. Was this how it would be until she died? Would we never be friends again? I couldn't swallow the pain this time. It was just too much.

Frank took me home, where I cried and cried, filled up a hot water bottle, took two Panadol and went to bed for a few hours. I remember Frank cooked scrambled eggs for dinner that night. We ate in silence in the smoke room. We couldn't talk at all. We didn't know what to say, really. We thought it best to let Tarry settle in in peace with just the medical staff around her. She was adamant that she wanted no contact with me at all.

I visited her again on Thursday afternoon, just two days before her 32nd birthday. She had quietened down, but she was not pleased to see me. I suggested a massage, but she would have none of that. I went home and Frank stayed on; she was happy to have her dad with her. This was to drive Frank and me apart for some considerable time, and Tarry knew it. She was becoming very manipulative.

On Friday, Tarry signed herself out of hospital and we didn't know where she had gone. After frantic phone calls we discovered she had arrived by taxi at Kristen's home. Frank drove straight over to bring her home here. If he had taken her back to Fairfield, she would probably have signed herself out again, unless she was certified as insane, and no one was prepared to do that. Not yet, anyway.

Kristen offered to care for her overnight and Tarry really wanted to stay with her. It was enough for us to know where she was and that she was safe. Kristen was very good with Tarry, who was in a highly-agitated state. The next morning, though, Tarry had left before Kristen woke up. It was Saturday, January 23, and Tarry's 32nd birthday. Kristen had no idea where she had gone. Once again we were on the phone, calling all her friends, trying to track her down.

Eventually we found her. She was at the home of a friend with whom she had traveled in South America all those years ago. This girl had put Tarry into bed, promising to take her back to Fairfield or to Kew, which was close by her home. She was not able to follow through with this, though. Another really reliable and wonderful friend of Tarry's took her home to her place in North Balwyn, where she comforted Tarry, kept her safe for the night and eventually cajoled her into returning to me.

I didn't see Tarry at all on her birthday. I cleared out of home and stayed out nearly all day. I bought a suit at Country Road and went by myself to see the film, *Enchanted April*.

I lost myself in that beautiful film. I wanted to block out the memory of 32 years ago, the day when Caroline was born and placed into my arms. I can still see her as she was then. She was the prettiest of all my babies. I loved holding her, and nursing her. I had just turned 23, and had such high hopes for my beautiful baby girl.

She hadn't let me down in any way. It was just that she was dying and I couldn't bear the thought of her leaving me forever, especially in a state of anger.

After the film ended, there was nothing to do but go home and wait to see what would happen next.

On Sunday morning at around 11:30, while Frank was still at Mass, Tarry, ashen-faced and subdued, came through the laundry door, took one look at me and burst into tears. I put my arms around her little shaking body and took her upstairs. I was so relieved to have her back with me. We sat together on the bed in my room and I rubbed her back to soothe her. I gave her my tiny gold and diamond ring, which I knew she had always admired. I had planned to leave it to her in my will.

She protested at first, saying she didn't deserve anything because she had caused so much trouble. I said it was a token of my love for her, past, present and future. I put it on her right-hand middle finger, and there it stayed always. Tarry was all smiles again, and so was I. We hugged each other close and shared together a precious magic moment of love and peace.

She agreed to return to Fairfield with me, where she was admitted to Ward 5. Frank collected her bag from Ward 4, and we waited on the bench outside her room while she settled in. She was calm and she was comfortable. Best of all, she was eager to be assessed properly and to resume taking her medication.

She was seen by a neurologist, who could find no evidence of a brain lesion, so it was concluded that her mental disturbances must be drug-instigated, and short of ceasing all AIDS medications, there was nothing that they could do about that. Having decided against discontinuing the medication, a mild tranquilizer was prescribed instead, and this seemed to help for a while. Tarry was also given a blood transfusion, for she had become quite anemic, and she had a colposcopy to see what stage the MAC was at. It was causing her great discomfort.

After a week in hospital, Tarry was discharged home to my care. We made all sorts of jellies, creme caramels and light puddings in our efforts to tempt her appetite. The wasting of her body was very evident now, although she was still quite strong on her feet.

In early February, Tarry was able to go to Portsea for a break with two of her closest friends. They waited on her hand and foot. The three of them, plus the two children of one of the friends, had a marvelous time together. Portsea is the most peaceful place on earth once the frantic holiday season has ended, and the weather is usually then at its best. It certainly was that February for Tarry and her friends.

Once home from Portsea, Tarry began to revert to an almost maniacal state. She was screaming and swearing and yelling at me day and night. She couldn't eat, and I was unable to handle her at all. I was at my wit's end. Nothing I said or did was right. She would taunt me, and laugh at me, and tell me I was useless. She said she had much more confidence in Frank and others who were much kinder to her. I think she was actually saying that she felt safer at Fairfield, and I can't say that I blame her for that. She began demanding on top note to be readmitted to Fairfield to have a naso-gastric tube introduced once more, in order to have the Ensure Plus feedings to nourish her. When Dominique came to help us with her on Monday night, February 15, she could see how desperate the situation had become.

Tarry was readmitted to Fairfield on Tuesday, February 16, 1993, and except for one weekend, she would never return home to live with us again. I had to face the fact that even though I was a nurse, and had cared for Tarry through the four years of her battle with AIDS, I was no longer able to provide the type of nursing care that she now needed. I was absolutely shattered. I felt a real failure now. I had lost her, swallowed up in a system full of computerized nursing management. I was exaggerating, of course, but I was full of rage, resentment and disappointment. All the while, though, I knew it was in Tarry's best interests for her to remain under the watchful eye of the wonderfully competent nursing staff, both male and female, who were so well trained in the care of AIDS patients. To their great credit, they were very understanding of my feelings, too.

When I arrived home from Fairfield, I looked up my ten guidelines again and felt reassured. We would all manage to cope if we remained calm and level-headed and in control.

Tarry spent a week in Ward Five, during which time she would ring up at night and hurl abuse at me, then ask to speak to her father. He would be asked for cigarettes, which were not obtainable at the hospital kiosk. She also wanted her car at Fairfield so she could take herself off-campus if she felt like it. Frank did provide the cigarettes, but he fixed the car up in such a way that she would never have access to it again. The car remained on the side lawn by the fence, under the English golden ash tree, until long after she had died. We eventually gave it to one of her friends who had done so much for her.

Each time I visited Tarry during those days, she would defiantly show me the door. So after one such episode, the next day I went to have my hair done instead of visiting her, and after that I made sure I had Margie or someone with me as a backstop. In a way I had become frightened of this foul-mouthed stranger who seemed hell-bent on giving me a hard time.

After one of her screaming bouts over the phone, I forgot my guidelines for goodness and peace. I snapped right there and then. I told her that she would die a lonely, friendless, unloved young woman if she didn't pull herself together, and consider the needs of others for a change (meaning me, of course). Frank was horrified as he overheard me delivering this speech. Tarry got a fright, though, and I was mighty glad I had said my piece. It was to be quite effective for a while.

On Tuesday, February 23, Jamie rang me from the Mercy Hospital birthing unit to say that Sally had been safely delivered of a son. Wonderful, wonderful news. The first Hurley grandson born to this generation. Jack Francis was his name. A wonderful, lusty lad, with powerful lungs which at brief and regular intervals he was only too pleased to entertain us with. He had the build of a boxer, and we all fell in love with him on the spot. Jack, like his cousin Greta, brought boundless golden joy into those dark gray days of my life. I only ever felt loving, loved, peaceful and needed when I held those two precious little babies in my arms.

On that same day, Tuesday, February 23, Tarry was transferred from Ward 5 to her new home in the Continuing Care Unit (CCU). It was a beautiful section of the hospital, devoted at this time to the respite care of AIDS patients. Her room in the unit was light and airy, with pretty curtains and a large window which overlooked the lawns and trees and the strutting peacocks with their peahens and little chicks.

Apart from Tarry, all the patients there were male. They all seemed to love her, both the staff and the patients. They understood her. They could see through and past all her ranting and raving and constant demands on their time and attention. They were always gentle, kind and loving towards Tarry. I will never forget their wonderful care of her.

Tarry became more and more demanding and aggressive, abrasive and messy in her dressing and habits. The nurse in charge of CCU explained that this was to be expected in AIDS patients and that I must not take it all to heart. It was no reflection on Caroline's upbringing, I was told. Well, thank God for small mercies, I thought.

But it was hard not to take all those horrible things to heart. I mean, Tarry was my daughter whom I had always loved and admired. After all, she was still my baby girl, no matter what age she was, and whatever she had turned into. I knew it was AIDS at work, but I couldn't stand what it was doing to her.

I took her favorite meals over to her each day, and for a while she really sparked up when she saw me coming. She asked for a wig. I got her one. She asked for new clothes to wear in her new home. I bought those, too. I massaged her each day, which I was very glad to do. I never, ever found that a chore. I also gave her my Swatch watch, as it had a large clear illuminated face and was easy for her to read. She always wanted to know what time it was.

After about a week of this fiercely demanding behavior, Tarry was reviewed by a psychiatrist, who prescribed an anti-psychotic drug for her. It was Haloperidol, or Serenace. It had the most appalling effect on Tarry. She became quite catatonic, lying almost in the fetal position, dribbling and drooling like an old lady in the advanced stages of senile dementia. We were all horrified.

Tarry was unable to speak and could barely hold a pen to scribble her needs on a little writing pad. Nor could she cough properly. Mucus and saliva collected at the back of her throat, so we all learned how to operate the bedside suction apparatus. It was a shocking sight and situation. Then, one night, a male nurse drew Dominique and me aside, to ask us if we knew who was bringing the drugs in for Tarry's use. "What drugs?" we said. What on earth was he talking about? We looked at each other totally perplexed. We didn't have the faintest idea what he was talking about.

On another day, I brought in some Oysters Kilpatrick, Tarry's favorite dish. I managed to help her sit up straight with the support of pillows. Her eyes lit up when she saw the oysters, but she was not able to eat them. Her trembling hand could not hold the little fork, which just slipped from her grasp and onto the bed. I speared an oyster for her and placed it into her mouth, which was all loose and slack. She was unable to swallow it. It just stayed in her mouth not moving one way or the other. I had to fish it out again in case it caused her to choke.

It was a frustrating and distressing experience, especially for Tarry. I couldn't believe that such a drastic drug would be prescribed for her, or perhaps it was the dosage that was drastic. I felt that I would rather have our Tarry back all ratty and unruly rather than have her in this state. Fortunately, the Haloperidol was ceased and Tarry came back to life again.

The days continued on as before. We brought in some meals when she felt she could manage them. She would ask for the re-use of the naso-gastric feeding on occasions. She walked with friends, family and other patients in the gardens, or tottered off to the kiosk for a cappuccino that was hardly ever consumed. She occasionally used her paints and sketch pad. Her friends arrived to take her on visits to other friends and restaurants, and during these times, the nursing staff tried to restore some order in her shambles of a room. Meanwhile, I took the washing and ironing home to attend to it.

I was becoming more and more frightened and frantic as Tarry became more wasted, restless and fearful. No one seemed to have any answers at all. But the gentleness, compassion and courtesy extended to Tarry and the family, especially to the almost constantly hysterically weeping mother, never wavered.

On Friday, March 12, Tarry was considered well and stable enough to come home for a weekend visit, complete with naso-gastric feeding in place. I was really pleased by this turn of events. I was planning a party for Jamie on the Sunday of that weekend, and some friends were joining us for lunch.

The friends were here from England on a business trip. A year ago we had made plans to accompany them on a four-day cruise around the Barrier Reef from Cairns to Cooktown to Lizard Island and back to Cairns. It would take six days in all, including the flight to Cairns from Melbourne and back again. We thought such a trip would now be impossible, but the CCU staff assured us that we should take this much-needed break away. They would watch over Tarry night and day. Our friends and Tarry's friends all rallied to encourage us to go. In the end, we agreed to take this holiday, for the situation was only going to become worse, much worse.

We brought Tarry home on Friday night. We arranged her comfortably on the smoke room couch in front of the TV. The plastic container of Ensure Plus was securely pinned to the curtains covering the windows beside her. Pillows were stacked around her for support.

The side effects of the Haloperidol were still apparent, even though the drug had not been administered for some days. Tarry walked with a strange, halting gait and there was a constant, involuntary twitching of her nose, as though it was itchy and she was unable to scratch it. I found out about those side effects by looking up a pharmaceutical medical dictionary which lists all approved drugs, their usage, dosage and dangers. So at least I knew what was causing these strange movements of Tarry's face and legs.

I helped loosen the tape that was holding the feeding tube in place, as Tarry was complaining that it was pulling on her skin. I cut off a new piece of tape to place over the tubing later. Tarry was watching the telly and sucking on a watery icy pole to keep her mouth moist. She looked miserable despite being surrounded by the comforts of home. I offered to take her up to bed, but she said she didn't feel tired and that she would stay up a bit later. I was very tired, though, so Frank said he would see her to bed.

I had much to do the following day in preparation for the Sunday lunch party for Jamie's birthday and the English friends. There would be 14 to cater for. I was so pleased that Tarry wanted to be with us once more, to join in a family gathering, in spite of being and feeling and looking so dreadfully ill. Her clothes now hung limply from her wasted little body. Each of her facial and skull bones stood out in stark relief. Her cheeks had sunken in as far as they could go – all the fatty tissue had dissolved away, leaving her skin stretched over the bones. Her teeth and gums were prominent, elongating her facial contours. She was taking on the appearance of a living skeleton. But the fire was still in her eyes, and that fire would burn right up until the end.

Early on Saturday morning I went into Tarry's room to reconnect the feeding tube, which we had agreed could be disconnected overnight to help her sleep more comfortably. Tarry was still sleeping peacefully, so I quietly reached up to start the machine. But there was nothing there and the tubing had all gone, too.

Tarry had cut through the tape and pulled out the tube. She had used the scissors I had the previous evening. I had left them, along with the roll of tape I had used, on the coffee table beside the couch. There was a tangled mess of tubing dangling over the side of the wastepaper bin beside her bed. She must have done this after everyone else had gone to bed that night. I was very annoyed about this but annoyance turned to horror, then fury, as I spied an empty blister pack of sleeping tablets caught up with the tubing.

She had tried to end her life by overdosing on "sleepers." I shook her shoulder and she stirred into wakefulness. I was furious. I ran from her room and immediately rang Tarry's doctor on her home number. Thank God she was still there. I told her what had happened, and after some discussion it was agreed that as Tarry was alright she could stay at home for the rest of the weekend if I felt I could manage her. I thought I could, so we left it at that for the present. Tarry had to return to Fairfield by six o'clock on Sunday evening, providing the situation remained stable.

Meanwhile, Frank had brought a cup of tea upstairs for us all, and had gone into Tarry's room to see what all the fuss was about. Tarry was crying now, saying that I was cross with her, and she wanted to go back to Fairfield immediately. I beckoned Frank out of the room and told him the story. He was shocked and terribly upset. In fact, I had never seen him so upset. I returned to her room and proceeded to tear strips off her. I had never before been so full of rage.

"How dare you do this to us," I yelled. "How could you even consider killing yourself like this, in the very bed that you slept in as a child, and in the home where you were brought up with all the care and love in the world? You rotten little wretch. How could you do this, and to your father of all people? How could you?" I was screaming at her now and she was crying.

"I'm sick of living with this disease. I just felt I couldn't go on any longer. I really didn't think about it much," croaked Tarry.

No sympathy was coming her way from me.

"I know you're sick of living, but we have all given every ounce of our beings to help you live – live with love all round you. Yet you, in one minute, would fling this all back in our faces, leaving us with even more grief, and feelings of guilt that we had failed you in some way."

I pointed out that if she had been some poor homeless, neglected girl who was left on her own to battle with AIDS, with no love to back her up, I just might consider helping her on her way. But for someone who had been protected, nurtured, worried about and loved so much, to consider such action was absolutely outrageous, wicked and cruel.

I have always been somewhat short-tempered, emotional and temperamental, but I really meant every word of this, and I do not regret saying it.

Then I burst into tears myself. I ran down the stairs and out the front door, fighting a rising feeling of hysteria. I could understand her desperation but I couldn't bear for her to die by her own hand. I begged God to help me help her see out the term of her natural life.

I remembered then that it was March 13, federal election day. *So what?* I thought. I got into the car, put on the sunglasses and drove to the polling booth at a local school. When I reached the head of the queue, a line was drawn through my name on the electoral role. To this day I have absolutely no idea for whom I voted. I just put a few numbers in a few squares, folded the paper and put it in the box and drove home again.

By now, Tarry was dressed and downstairs looking in the fridge for something soft to eat. She had settled down and so had I. She made me promise not to tell the staff at CCU. That was easy to agree to because I had already told her doctor, who would have passed the information on by now.

I told Tarry that we would draw up a list of foods that she must eat every hour, on the hour. A lightly boiled egg, a small cup of Milo, a little dish of ice cream or custard and jelly. She kept valiantly to this routine all Saturday and most of Sunday. I still have that list of foods that she forced herself to eat that day. She really seemed to be sorry for what she had done.

I still had all the work to do for the lunch next day. It was to be a simple meal: salad Nicoise and a variety of crusty breads, and the inevitable tira-mi-su, which fell apart when I turned it out onto the large platter. I swore, and stuck it together with extra marscapone cheese and covered it with cocoa powder and berries. It looked quite presentable as I tucked it away in the fridge again.

I set the table in the dining room with a long white damask cloth, and Tarry helped me with the cutlery. She picked ivy for me to put with the other greenery on the table center. I wrote out name cards and placed them strategically, so that, hopefully, everyone would communicate happily with those around them. I placed Tarry's card next to her father at the head of the table. She was very pleased about that. She forgot about it the next day and complained to Dominique that I had not set a place for her at the table at all!

The harder I worked during that day, the less time I spent dwelling on Tarry's latest episode. I didn't tell the others until after Sunday was over. Tarry slept most of that day, and Saturday night as well. She was rather grumpy on Sunday morning, but I was too busy to pay her much attention.

I was proud of her performance that Sunday. She really rose to the occasion and was natural and friendly to all, as they were to her. Two of our English friends had known Tarry for many years and had always admired her beauty and bouncy personality. They showed no shock, just love and affection when they met her once again.

The day was a great success, and this was due largely to Tarry's courageous courtesy. It was a really special and happy day, although by the end of it I was absolutely exhausted from hiding the strain of the previous day's events. I was glad when six o'clock came and we could take Tarry back to Fairfield. I went straight to bed and, for a change, slept reasonably well.

Dominique told me later that all during that Sunday afternoon Tarry had pestered her and her boyfriend, Margie and Peter and Kristen for money to buy drugs to kill herself. She had left Jamie alone because it was his birthday. They didn't give her any money, but they knew what she had done, and they were amazed that Frank and I could get through the day without falling apart. So were we.

The children were very upset by her requests for money, but I felt reasonably sure that she would be unlikely to try to take her life again. It had been a great shock to us all, and we said nothing about it to anyone, not anyone at all.

The next two days saw quite an improvement in Tarry psychologically. I think that she was very grateful that we had stopped being cross with her, and she was feeling secure and happy in the environment of CCU. The staff had redoubled their efforts to persuade us to fly off to Cairns on Thursday. They were adamant that after all the recent drama, we should take a break.

We did go, and we had a wonderful few days. We felt free, free from responsibility. We laughed and played with our English friends during those sparkling tropical days and languid evenings, with the cruiser sailing along in constantly smooth waters.

As we flew home to Melbourne on Thursday, March 25, the fear returned with us. We went straight home from the airport, rang Tarry, and said we would be right over. "Good," she said, and would her father bring a Paddle Pop ice cream? The shops were shut, I told her. She seemed annoyed by this, but we were so anxious to see her that we didn't stop to look for any milk bars that might still have been open.

Tarry greeted us with open arms when we arrived in her room. Apparently she had done nothing but talk about our coming home since the day we left. She was delighted with the little opal ring we had bought for her at a market held weekly in the hotel complex on the waterfront in Cairns. It was really too big for her, but she insisted on wearing it. I noticed that her tummy had become very swollen, which emphasized the extreme thinness of the rest of her body.

She told us that there had been at least two deaths in CCU while we were away. She also told us how helpful she had been with making cups of tea for the grieving relatives. I wondered about that, although in a way it did not surprise me, for she had always been very practical when others faced times of trouble, and she still did not seem to see herself as one approaching her own death.

She was booked for another CAT scan of her stomach on Friday, March 26, the following day, and this time Frank volunteered to drive her out to Moreland. He set out for Fairfield that day with the requested Paddle Pops, new leggings, jumper and scarf. I was pleased to buy these smart new clothes for her. She never wore a nightie during the day at the hospital. She was always dressed in "street" clothes, so I had to keep her supply of them up to the mark. She made a terrible mess of them, with melted icy poles, spilt coffee, cigarette ash and so on.

She was wearing children's size clothes now. Baggy pants over the tights to hide her matchstick legs, scarves to protect her neck from draughts, and wooly hats pulled down around her face. Long, roomy jumpers completed the outfit. She was indeed a travesty of the truly beautiful girl she had once been. But she hung onto her dignity and pride. She was still our dearly beloved daughter.

On Saturday, March 27, Tarry seemed bright and happy and wanted to come home. She wanted to see Enchanted April, followed by a roast beef dinner before returning to Fairfield. Frank and I thought this would be wonderful.

But it was a disaster. We had to bring her home early from the film. She was restless and irritable in the theater and was disturbing the other patrons. She picked at the roast beef and then demanded to return to hospital. She wanted to be with her friends, she said. So back she went to Fairfield and we, dejected, came home to bed.

The next day Tarry's wonderful friends, the "card girls," picked her up from the hospital, with permission, of course, and drove her to a friend's home in Geelong, an hour southwest of Melbourne, for the day. She had a wonderful time, but was very difficult with them too. She wanted to stop at the bank, then she asked for take-away food, which when bought, she didn't, or couldn't, eat. It was apparent to the "card girls" also that this was all part of the mental deterioration process that came courtesy of the AIDS virus.

This went on from day to day, and no one knew what would happen next. My whole world revolved around Tarry at this time. I managed to play the occasional game of bridge, have the hair done, and had frequent blessed visits from the grandchildren and their mothers. Darling Greta and Jack restored my flagging spirits every time they came into the house.

Without realizing it, I was becoming very thin myself. I was often bone weary and would forget to eat. It was the hairdresser who pointed out how thin I was. He told me that I should be taking better care of myself. He was never one to mince his words, but he was right. I ate more Cornettos, and the sugar fix did the trick. I used to love Cornettos as much as Tarry did, but now that she is no longer here to eat them with me, I can't face them any more. As well as eating ice creams, I put my massage practice on hold for a while, to give myself a rest; I really was exhausted.

More trouble was brewing. I discovered that Tarry had been asking friends for money, friends who could ill afford to meet those demands. One girl was particularly distressed by Tarry's manipulative ways, and was forced to tell me about it. I reimbursed her and reassured her. She must not visit Tarry again for both their sakes, I told her. She had to look after her own life and well-being. She loved Tarry, but she could no longer cope with her. It was so sad for her to have to let go. They had been friends since school days. Tarry asked after her friend once or twice and then she appeared to forget her. I rang around the rest of her friends to find that she had been asking them for money as well, but none had been given to her.

Tarry's demands for anything and everything were made on each member of the family. In a hoarse, strident pitch and tone quite alien to her normal voice, she would insist on instant gratification of her wishes. All this was beginning to get on everyone's nerves. However, remarkable patience was demonstrated by all and sundry. We all knew that this was AIDS talking and not our true Tarry. There were times, though, when it was all too much.

On one particular afternoon at the hospital there was a real showdown. Tarry had been nagging away at one of her sisters: "Get my cigarettes, lighter, matches, Fanta, Paddle Pop, red icy pole. Now!" No please or thank you, just "Get it!"

Her sister, under great duress, exploded. "What would your Royal Highness like now? More cigarettes, lighters, more icy poles, perhaps? Yes sir! Yes sir! Three bags full sir!" she shrieked on top note at Tarry, who looked very taken aback.

Tarry's reply, in a little girl, petulant voice was "I'm just a poor sick girl. You'll be sorry when I die!"

"Don't bet on it, sweetheart," replied her sister, *sotto voce*. The poor girl then burst into tears and ran out of the room. It was all so terrible for the two suffering sisters, and for those looking on.

They both needed love and reassurance Tarry because she was so ill, and could not help what she was doing or saying, and her sister because she felt so ashamed and guilty for losing her patience with her. There is no place for guilt on these occasions; all behavior was quite understandable and very normal. They settled down again after much cuddling, back patting and a big kiss each.

Such an occurrence was a very isolated one throughout the whole of Tarry's illness. When all is said and done, we are all human and there are natural limits to our patience and tolerance. I have no reservations writing about this short episode, however stressful it appears. I know the depths of the love and affection that all members of the family felt for and extended to Tarry. And I also know that the same was reciprocated by Tarry, and to an equal degree. She was never to feel any sense of rejection by her family — a fate so commonly, and so cruelly, suffered by so many afflicted with this dreadful disease.

One Sunday afternoon in early April, Tarry spent the day at home with me. She seemed quite normal and happy. I had become used to her constant demands, which were par for the course now, and I had learned to distract her attention from some of those demands simply by changing the topic of conversation instantly. She chatted away happily about this and that, and we were very comfortable together. It was wonderful to feel close to her even for a little while.

Little more than an hour after I had returned her to CCU, though, she was on the phone screaming abuse at me once more. Her boyfriend had stolen $1000 from her and she would speak only to Frank. She was hysterical. It turned out that the preceding Friday, the "boy wonder" had taken Tarry to her bank by taxi and there she had signed several withdrawal slips, enabling him to access the invalid pension money in her account. Every fortnight, it seems, when Tarry's cheque had been paid in, he used to cycle along to the bank and withdraw the money, which apparently would be shot straight up his arm. It was true that he loved Tarry, but now he was locked in the loveless arms of heroin. Frank calmed Tarry down, arranged to have power of attorney over her affairs, and the money stopped disappearing from her bank account.

With that mess sorted out, we now planned to have Tarry at home with us on Easter Sunday, April 11. I thought this year, weather permitting, we would have a picnic lunch outside by the pool, and to my delight, the weather permitted. It was a superb, mild sunny day. I had cooked and prepared every single one of Tarry's favourite dishes and spread them out on a green and white checked cloth on the breakfast room table. Easter eggs were dotted among the dishes and platters. It all looked wonderful. I was hoping that Tarry would think so, too.

She arrived at lunchtime with friends of hers: a young couple and their children who were very fond of her. Tarry had been very good to them in troubled times, and they were more than willing to help care for her now in her time of agonizing need for love and understanding.

Tarry hobbled through the house and out into the garden, by the pool; there she collapsed, exhausted, onto a sun lounge in the shade. I was hoping that she would not see her car on the other side of the pool fence, and demand to drive it. She didn't even notice it was there. To please me, she tried to eat a little of the food. She realized it had all been done for her, but she just couldn't manage it. She tried to drink a small glass of beer, but she later vomited this up.

We all sat around her chatting, while the children played in the pool. She looked so sad and little lying there. All afternoon I watched her as she looked wistfully around the garden, at the trees, the roses in the rockeries, and at the house as though she might never see them this way again.

She had appreciated my efforts to please her, but by the time five o'clock arrived she was desperate to return to her home, her room in CCU, Fairfield. She was always a little bit brighter when she returned to the hospital. It was neutral ground for her there. It was a "home" that held no past or future. It was a here-and-now place of living and security that made it easier for her to loosen the ties that bound her to us.

In a sense Tarry regarded her fellow patients in the continuing care unit as her other and more personal family. She spent hours talking to them, sometimes when they were in their very last stages. She comforted them, and they her. She would refer to each of them by name and call each of them "my friend." This fulfilled one of the aims of Fairfield Hospital in establishing the CCU. It was to provide another "home" for the patients in the late stages of AIDS. As in a home, the bed or room was kept for each patient even if he or she was elsewhere for two or three nights. A secondary object was to provide some respite for the outside carers by supplying intermittent short stays in the unit. It resulted in a variation of routine for the sufferers and some rest for the outside carers. It was unique and it was wonderful.

CHAPTER 12

⟡

THE TIDE RUNS OUT

April drew to a close and we headed into early May, and with each passing day Tarry continued to deteriorate in spite of her enormous efforts to keep on the move. She still went out at night with her friends when she felt well enough. She had permission to do this, of course. They carried her or took along a wheelchair when she could no longer walk. She struggled out to see bands, or visit restaurants with friends where she would order large, mainly Asian meals, which she left untouched.

She no longer cared about her medications. Both at home and in hospital, tablets would be discovered under pillows, in pockets, under the bed, in bedside drawers. The pill-taking was rarely supervised and even if it was, Tarry would sometimes just hold the tablets in her mouth, then spit them out again when no one was looking. She told me about this with the secretive giggling attitude of an errant schoolgirl.

One day when Tarry was out on a visit something really beautiful happened for her. A friend of Margie had posted a parcel to Tarry. It was waiting for her on her bed in her freshly tidied up room in CCU. Tarry read the accompanying letter first.

The sender had gone out into her country garden early in the morning and had run around catching autumn leaves before they reached the ground. When gathered this way by someone for somebody else, these leaves were said to have magic powers. All these magic leaves had been parceled up for Tarry to strengthen her hope and love and peace of mind. Tarry was enthralled by this legend, as was everyone else.

One of the nurses attached each leaf to the large window beside Tarry's bed. There they stayed until Tarry died. They never fell to the ground, or floor, and were a constant source of delight to Tarry and her many visitors. Their presence did seem to make her more peaceful. She loved flowers and she received so many of them, brought in by her friends and ours, all during her time in hospital.

She became weaker and weaker. Each day and evening one or more of her sisters or her brother would arrange to be with her, and her friends were always close by, too. Kristen was marvelous. She seemed to be more available than the others. Not having family commitments left her freer to visit in the evenings. She would sit with Tarry for hours on end, just keeping her company. "After all," said Kristen, "we never did have much to say to each other, so we are hardly likely to keep up a running conversation now."

She was right, of course. She sat with her knitting as she watched over her sister. This was especially good in the awful hour after twilight when darkness descends. It is the most depressing time for people when they are ill.

I had been made aware that Tarry had been referring to death from time to time – not her own death, apparently, but death in general. She had not broached the subject with me at all in recent times. It seemed she had never talked the topic through with anyone, and I had the feeling that Tarry really knew she was dying and desperately needed to be prepared for this next huge and final journey.

She had formed a great rapport with the Catholic hospital chaplain, but not as yet to the point of discussing death. This wonderful man had listened to her tell of her traveling days and her unusual life experiences. He realized that, in essence, Tarry was an intensely spiritual person, with a great love of a universal God; her spirituality encompassed many faiths, including Catholicism, but not exclusively so. She and I used to agree that the Catholic Church had not "cornered the market" on God. With great patience, compassion and wisdom, this priest gently encouraged her conversations with him.

He was so kind to me, too, when I fell into a real trough of grief some weeks before Tarry's death. I was constantly bursting into tears as I arrived at the hospital each day. Father Peter suggested that it might be better all round if I stopped visiting Tarry, as it seemed to be distressing me to the point of becoming sick myself. After all, he pointed out, I wouldn't be able to visit if I really were sick, so why make myself sick? What a gentle, subtle way of releasing me from my ties at Fairfield. I actually did stay away for one day, during which I calmed down and reached a decision. It was going to be up to me to tell Tarry that she was dying, and to help her prepare for this, as carefully and gently as I could.

It was a terrifying task to face. I was afraid I would stir up her angry feelings towards me again; but it had to be done, and I knew that I was the only person who could do it. Frank agreed with me. Tarry had always trusted me during her years with AIDS. We had endured so much together with great mutual respect and love, tears and laughter, and now we were silently sharing a good measure of fear. There had been so many rows and fights between us during the past four months, but they had ceased for now at least. Time was quickly running away from us. We could not afford to procrastinate. I could not, and would not, let her die in anger, fear and frustration.

On Sunday, May 9, we celebrated Margie's 30th birthday and Mother's Day with a small family lunch at Kew. We brought Tarry home to be with us. I set the table for eight in the sunlit family room. Autumn leaves were scattered as decoration across the round white tablecloth. Tarry was taken with all this and the family togetherness.

A wonderful atmosphere of peace prevailed as the eight of us sat down to lunch. Tarry couldn't eat, but she held Greta in her arms while the rest of us tucked in. Soon, she handed Greta back to her mother, and lay down to rest on the couch beside the dining table. She slept while we had coffee and birthday cake.

My decision had now been made: the following day at Fairfield, I would speak to Tarry about her approaching death. I felt terribly sick and anxious. While I cleared up the kitchen later in the afternoon, Margie, Peter and Greta drove Tarry back to CCU and settled her in. As I went about my chores, I tried to work out the best way in which to tackle tomorrow's task.

In the early afternoon of Monday, May 10, I drove out to Fairfield, shaking with apprehension. On arriving, I went into Tarry's room, and there she was, sitting up on a chair beside her bed, looking ghastly. She was quite chirpy, though, in the midst of the shambles of paints and brushes and canvases, untouched food, cigarette stubs and two half-drunk bottles of Fanta.

She seemed very pleased to see me and said so. That was a great relief for me. We linked arms and she leaned against me as we wobbled our way around to the balcony room. I had suggested that we sit there. It was a lovely quiet, sunlit area, overlooking another aspect of the Fairfield gardens and had soft easy chairs placed in groups around small tables. It was warm and some way away from the smoking area. It was a very suitable area for a private conversation, or just to sit and be quiet.

There was no chapel at the hospital at that time. There is one now, and it will soon be fully completed for the use of all patients of all faiths. It is a wonderful addition in the provision of total patient care; their spiritual needs will surely be satisfied in this lovely new environment.

Tarry made herself comfortable in the lounge chair and I sat opposite her. I had brought with me my kit of scented oils and towels so that I could massage Tarry's feet and legs while we talked. It would also give me something to do, a sort of secondary purpose for being there if the original project fell flat. I lifted her bare feet onto a folded towel on my lap and rolled up the legs of her soft tracksuit pants. As I started the massage we were chatting about Margie's birthday and how good Greta had been during the afternoon.

Then Tarry told me that one of the patients had died in CCU yesterday while Tarry had been at Kew. At least, she thought it was yesterday. She wasn't sure. Her mind was beginning to drift away. I had to bring it back, for this was the perfect moment to talk about her death. Without looking at her, I asked Tarry if she had given any thought to the possibility that her own death was approaching. She said that she had, but she did not wish to talk about it. My heart was racing as I said that was fine and went back to concentrating on rhythmically massaging her feet.

After a while I looked up at her. She was looking at me very intensely, her eyes wide and round.

"When do you think I will die, Mum?" she asked.

"I'm not sure, darling," I said, "but I think it could be very soon, perhaps two weeks or two months, but you really are dying."

As I said this to her, I actually began to feel quite calm, and my heart slowed down. This was going to be alright. It seemed almost natural to be talking with Tarry like this. She appeared to be quite relaxed, as well. This is a miracle, I thought.

I then asked her if she would like to tell me about her concept of death, or rather life after death. What might she expect to experience? She replied that she would like to discuss this with me, but first she wanted to hear what I thought about life after death.

This was quite an easy task for me. I did not believe in the old Catholic concept of heaven with which we had been indoctrinated at school. Neither did Tarry, and we did not believe in hell at all. I told Tarry that I had always believed that Nanna and Auntie Vera would be waiting for me when I died. They would greet me, welcome me into the next life and keep me safe. I really believed this, and I still do. I suggested to Tarry that as she was apparently going to die before me, did it make any sense to her that her beloved Nanna and Auntie Vera would be waiting for her ahead of me?

She was delighted with that idea. It certainly did make sense to her. It was something to believe in – a real and positive idea that she could actually look forward to. What she didn't actually put into words was the fact that now she felt able to let go; she was "allowed" to die. She was more afraid of the actual process of dying than death itself, she told me.

I knew I could help her deal with these fears. I promised her faithfully that she would not die alone or lonely. I would be right beside her, holding her and loving her, as would her father, and hopefully her sisters and brother, whom she loved so much, just as they had always loved her. We would all be there to care for her right to the end. I really begged God to hear my plea, and make this all come true. He did, as it turned out. I also promised her that she would not die in pain; no physical or emotional pain would touch her. No pain of any kind would interfere with her preparation for her last great journey into her new life beyond this world.

We were so close at that moment. I will never forget it, and it comforts me still whenever I feel sad, missing my Tarry. She remained peaceful, calm and relaxed. The fear and anxiety had left her face, and her lovely eyes looked dreamlike. She smiled at me and we had a big hug.

By this stage, I had forgotten about her feet, which were resting in my lap and feeling rather cold. I friction-rubbed them warm again, replaced the pink lambswool slippers and went to the kitchen to make us a cup of tea. I was feeling quite amazed, really. I had achieved what I had set out to do, and Tarry still loved and trusted me after all. I didn't know then that more nightmares were to occur in the short time that we had Tarry left to us.

I kissed Tarry goodbye and saw her back to her room. By this stage, she was very tired, and quite agitated once again, and was asking for painkillers. I told a trusted staff member what had been going on and drove home, absolutely exhausted. I could hardly walk through the back door into the kitchen, where I could see Frank waiting for me.

He made me sit down while I told him what had happened. He had been so anxious himself during the past three hours. It was now four o'clock in the afternoon. He said he was proud of me. I liked that. Then he helped me upstairs to have a rest.

I fell asleep for a while, and when I woke I carefully went over the events of that afternoon. Perhaps it was God who had inspired me to say the right thing at the right time. Maybe Tarry's death really would be safe and peaceful after all.

We learned from the chaplain the next day that Tarry had happily received the Sacrament of the Sick and Holy Communion. This was symbolic of the rituals before death encompassing all religious beliefs. Tarry had re-entered the faith into which she had been baptized. She had obviously given this much thought and we were all so happy for her. She was part of the spiritual system of the universe once more.

Tarry continued on her merry way, determined to squeeze every ounce of action out of the time that was left to her. She found ways of going out and planned all kinds of unmanageable activities. The "card girls" came to the rescue with a wonderful idea that was to make Tarry feel very special and in charge. They asked if they could come to Kew on the evening of Thursday, May 13. They would bring the food and drinks and have a little "card girls" gathering, with Tarry acting as hostess.

Tarry was beside herself with this idea. I bought her a whole new outfit: a long woolen wrap-around green skirt, matching ribbed loose-fitting polo-necked jumper, a floppy velour beret, and also matching warm woolen tights. Her friends wheeled her through the front door, all dressed up, looking absolutely appalling, an uncertain smile on her face. My heart ached for her.

Unperturbed, her friends all fussed around her. They all settled themselves in the family room. Drinks were poured, food was laid out, the music blared and the laughter rang out. I left them to it. It was their night, not mine. Margie was there to help. She had brought Greta with her to keep Frank and me amused and occupied.

There were some tears mixed with the laughter that night, but all in all, it was a great success. Two of the girls carried Tarry upstairs, undressed her and put her to bed in her own room once more. They all said their goodbyes and made happy plans to return on the following Thursday.

After seeing the girls off, I returned upstairs to Tarry and all hell let loose. She began yelling and swearing at me for not having her sleeping pills ready for her. I had already given them to her with a drink of water. She eventually went to sleep and I just turned away and went to bed myself. But this latest outburst from Tarry made it difficult for me to sleep.

The next morning Tarry was very contrite, but I really didn't care. I was too damned tired. Frank carried her downstairs. She loved being carried, she told him, and nestled into his shoulder. No breakfast was eaten, just a mouthful of orange juice. We drove back to Fairfield, mainly in silence, each of us occupied with our own thoughts.

Tarry was quite calm now. She told us she had reached a decision. She wanted to be taken off all AIDS medication and to be given only pain relief and "sleepers." Frank and I spoke about this at length with the doctors involved. After telling us the possible consequences of this action, which were that she might succumb more quickly to infection, they agreed to cease medication. I thanked the doctors, especially Tarry's own doctor, who had cared for her for so long and lovingly. I thanked them for services so generously and kindly rendered, and almost joyfully I returned to Tarry to tell her that her wish had been granted.

She, too, was pleased that the medical hold on her AIDS-ridden life was being relinquished. Nothing further could be done for her to improve the quality of her life, a life she had lived so courageously and well. It would soon be time for her to leave it behind, and until that time the only medication to be given would be to keep Tarry free of pain and comfortably asleep at night.

Tarry now began making rather bizarre plans to leave hospital as soon as she was "well enough." She wished to begin a new life with one of her dearest friends. This girl was so kind and caring. She even had the courtesy to consult me about this little charade, in case it might upset me. We encouraged Tarry with her plans, which we all knew would never eventuate.

In a way, it seemed to me that the new life being planned at her friend's home was really a kind of anticipation of her imminent death and passage to her true new life. Tarry promised that she would visit me frequently at home. She was so happy and relieved that I did not expect her to live at Kew with me again.

I felt wretched, though. It seemed that I too had become a kind of symbol of death to Tarry. We had talked so intimately of her death. She knew that I knew she would soon be dead. I was even beginning to wish I had said nothing. I felt very lonely and rejected.

Everybody else seemed to be doing a much better job of caring for Tarry. While very friendly to others, she was only formally pleasant toward me. Perhaps I was imagining this. I didn't know what to do. Once again I drove down to Portsea by myself to reassess the situation. I would have another look at those 10 guidelines or commandments. They needed a bit of adjusting perhaps.

I went for a walk along the Portsea back beach, where I renewed my promise to Tarry to scatter her ashes from London Bridge. I was crying and crying with fatigue, frustration and fear. Fortunately there was no one around me. I resolved to make an appointment to see the wonderful psychiatrist from those early days. I could unload my doubts and fears onto him. I also resolved not to let the interference we were encountering from some of the relatives get me down as much as it had. After all, I was Caroline's mother, and it was unfair to be walked over and made to feel inadequate and resentful. There was no time for negative feelings now.

I felt better when I arrived back at the house but not for long, however, for there were more shocks in store for me.

I had already begun to collect my things to pack into the car for my return to Melbourne when I glanced through the living room window at the late autumn sun shining on the lawn and trees. It looked so peaceful and inviting, I thought I would go outside and rest in it for a while before driving home. I opened the front door, then the screen door and went to step out in my bare feet onto the veranda. As I did so, I looked down, and there on the doormat was a headless, freshly disembowelled rat. I jumped back into the room, slammed the door and went to pieces.

I screamed and screamed. I was totally hysterical. I believed that someone had put that hideous thing there, as some kind of curse or part of a strange satanic ritual, a ritual that in some disgusting way involved me. The dear old man from the house next door came running across the lawn. He saw what was on the doormat, and stepping over this abomination, he came inside and put his arms around me to try to calm me down. When eventually he had succeeded, he reassured me and explained that it was nothing more sinister than the work of a local cat. He then set to and disposed of all the horrible bits and pieces, and hosed down the veranda.

I will never forget Brian for his wonderful kindness to me on that day. He offered to take me back to his home to have dinner with him and his wife, but I felt too sick and shivery to eat, or do anything else, either. Instead of driving back to Melbourne as planned, I filled up a hot water bottle and went to bed. I was too frightened to move, and had nightmares all night about that rat.

Next morning, I woke up exhausted. I made up my mind to keep the events of the previous day to myself. There was nothing to be gained by telling such a tale of horror at such a time. I had told Frank, of course, as that was why I had not gone back to Kew the previous evening. I rested for a few more hours, had something to eat and drink and thought about my revised resolutions once more. Then feeling calmer and a bit more reasonable, I drove back to Melbourne.

As soon as I was back in Kew, Sunday, May 23, Frank and I went straight out to Fairfield to bring Tarry home for the night. She had been worried about me, she said, as she had heard that I was upset. She could hardly move she was so weak, so Frank carried her to the car. We drove slowly home to Kew. We all felt sure it would be for the last time.

Once at home, we settled Tarry on the couch in the smoke room. She was supported by soft pillows and covered with a rug. A hot water bottle warmed her aching back. The three of us were to share a wonderful, warm, loving evening together. I loved being able to hold Tarry close to me again. She leaned her head against my chest as we all watched The House of Eliott. We loved that program. Such beautiful clothes and the upstairs-downstairs atmosphere had great appeal. Tarry tried to tackle a Cornetto as she watched the telly, but she couldn't manage it at all. We kept her mouth moist by giving her large lemon-flavored cottonbuds to suck. All loneliness, fear and frustration just melted away that evening, thank God. And we had Tarry overnight with us this one last time.

We returned Tarry to Fairfield on Monday morning, whereupon I began clearing the clutter from her hospital room. I didn't touch those autumn leaves, of course. I packed up the clothing that she would no longer require. Her paints, paintings and books were stacked into large plastic bags, and I took all of this home. She had no further use for them and she no longer cared about them. I took everything back to Kew.

As I sorted through all these things belonging to Tarry, I felt quite calm. Some items that had been pilfered by her were returned to their owners. Other things I threw away. Keepsakes I gave away. I put all of Tarry's real treasures aside to distribute among family members, and her close friends. Her little bottle of perfume from Morocco I gave to her godmother. Some treasures I kept for Frank and myself to touch and reminisce over in the days, months and years to come. They rekindle such happy memories of the wonderful life she had before the onset of AIDS. Tarry's quaint Mexican clothing and costumes were bundled off to the dry cleaners. They have been stored away for "dress-ups" for the grandchildren as they grow older. I was glad to do all this before Tarry died. It made for a lighter burden to carry afterwards. The idea was given to me by a very wise woman, and I am so glad that I followed her advice.

By Wednesday, May 26, Tarry was really dying. She was in the full throes of pneumonia and was lapsing in and out of consciousness. Oxygen and suction were helping her to breathe. She was in no pain; the automatic administration of regular doses of morphine from a syringe carefully strapped to her chest ensured this. She had no fear. There was peace and solace all around her, and she had the company of those she felt comfortable with. All through the day, her brother, sisters and other family members called in one by one. They sat by her bed, touching her, holding back their tears and playing her favorite music on the cassette recorder on her bedside table. Her room was pleasantly and delicately perfumed by an aromatherapy vaporizer that was lit on her windowsill, just under the autumn leaves.

The nursing care Tarry received was excellent. The nurses amazed me, they were so courteous and compassionate, so young to be faced with deaths of people their own age group on an almost daily basis. At regular intervals everything that needed to be done to maintain her comfort was carried out with the greatest care and tenderness. She was always comfortably positioned in a clean nightie, with fresh white sheets and large soft pillows. Her old teddy bear sat gazing down at her from his perch at the top of the pillow.

All I did was sit there looking on. I felt as though I was dreaming. All Thursday and Thursday night, I sat on one side of her bed, with Frank on the other, and Kristen there also. She watched over Tarry in her delirium while I slept for a while on the next bed. Tarry was burning with fever, and at the same time she was asking for a party and a new party dress. By 10:30 pm we did not think that she would survive the night. But Tarry would surprise everybody.

When Tarry was in Tibet all those years ago, she had acquired an inkpad and stamp which spelled her name in Tibetan characters. Well, this is what she believed, anyway. In hospital, she kept the stamp, with its inkpad, beside her on her locker. She was so proud of it. So when three of her "card girl" friends paid her a surprise visit at 11:00 pm on this sad, sad night, we all put stamps on the backs of our hands to help the "party" atmosphere along. Tarry was excited and delighted by this: it was as though a special club had been formed in her honor, and the "Tarry tats" were the symbol that one belonged to this exclusive little club. Where she had appeared to be almost unconscious half an hour earlier, the change when the girls walked in even before they had spoken was quite astonishing.

The "card girls" stayed with Tarry until one o'clock the following morning. When they kissed their old friend goodbye and left, they were in tears, and so were we. They knew they would never see her again, and they had loved her so much, for so many years.

Frank and I left Tarry's room at 4:00 am. It was now Friday, May 28, Tarry's last full day on this earth.

Later that morning Margie and I decided to buy Tarry a real party dress. We went to Ishka in High Street, Kew, where we bought a really beautiful gown: long and crimson, all velvet and chiffon with soft, sheer, floating sleeves that came to the elbow. We also bought some bright-colored bead necklace strands, and to complete the outfit, a little satin bag.

We raced back to Fairfield with our special purchases, and Tarry was delighted with them. She was quite lucid now. She chatted weakly as we slipped the wondrous party dress over her head, neck and arms, draping the long skirt over the bedspread. As the beads were placed around her neck, Tarry wore a look of enthrallment. The little satin bag was held loosely in her fingers.

Tarry remained conscious and close to me for most of that day. I cuddled her and covered her head and face with the kisses she craved. I massaged her hands and feet, but did so very gently. She got all the love and reassurance that I had to give. She was peaceful, and I could see that she was happy.

On that Friday evening I was able to leave the family to have dinner on their own while I spent two whole hours with Tarry, just the two of us. This was possible thanks to the kindness of our wonderful, caring friends who kept Kew on the go with generous supplies of delicious casseroles and other good things. They knew that I was at Fairfield nearly all the time now, and they helped out in the most thoughtful and practical ways. I was so grateful to them, for I had no thoughts other than being with Tarry.

Apart from the recent disturbances, Tarry and I had always had a great rapport, especially over these last years and when we had traveled together, all those years ago. In many ways, I had envied her seemingly breezy lifestyle and adventurous spirit. Had I been younger, I feel sure I would have been tempted to live like she did just a little bit. We both hated and regretted the conflict that the accursed AIDS had caused to rage between us from time to time. But now, all conflict was over, completely gone, and we were so peaceful and full of love once more.

As I held her close to me that night, she told me things about herself that I had never known, or perhaps had only guessed at. She knew this would clear up a number of mysteries about the life she had led over the last decade. She also knew that she could trust me to remain silent, which I have.

Tarry asked me to keep holding her and stroking her. She had always loved me, she said, and she thanked me for loving and understanding her, adding that she was very glad she hadn't succeeded in killing herself. She was so sorry she had caused me such pain. I was so touched by that. I had loved being her mum so much. My heart was truly breaking at the thought of her leaving me behind.

I couldn't hide the tears any longer as I placed Nanna's and Auntie Vera's rosary beads around her neck and watched Tarry thread them through her fingers with a smile. She was happy that she would soon be scattered over the sea. Death no longer held any fears for my Tarry. She was guaranteed a safe entry into the next life.

> And in the midst of all our pain and grief
> I held my daughter, lighter than a leaf.
> When Caroline looked up into my face
> I saw again her beauty and her grace.

Frank arrived soon after this. I left them alone for a while, and then we waited for Tarry to settle. We went home at 11:30 pm, praying that she would not die before our return in the morning.

We hurried back to Fairfield early on Saturday morning. Kristen arrived soon after. Tarry was now very close to death. Her breathing was light and shallow, a little pulse throbbed in her neck. Her eyes were half closed and glazed, but I thought I could detect a little light left in them.

A very kind young nurse asked me if I would like to sponge-bathe Tarry for the very last time. I was more than happy to be able to do this. I had missed out on so much of her actual nursing care in these last months. Together the nurse and I slipped the sweat-soaked nightie off

Tarry's tiny, wasted body. I washed her ever so gently and we carefully turned her onto her other side and placed another fresh nightie over her. She sighed and settled back on the pillows.

Tarry was only just conscious, but she was able to communicate with a faint nod, and a feathery touch of her fingers on the back of my hand. Frank and Kristen stroked her thin little arms while I cuddled her head on my shoulder. The scented vaporizer candle kept burning and the Gregorian Chant, Tarry's favorite music for some time, was softly playing in the background. She was surrounded by love, warmth and peace.

The gaps between each breath became longer. Tarry nodded when I asked her if she could see Nanna and Auntie Vera. I said we would now take her to them and after that we would have a great big party in her honor to celebrate the beginning of her greatest adventure ever. We would then take her to Portsea for a long, long rest, and one day we would all be with her again, all of us together.

Tarry nodded again, sighed a little shallow sigh and stopped breathing. She was dead. It was 1:10 pm exactly on Saturday, May 29, 1993, and I could not believe it. She was actually gone from me forever. How could I ever get used to not having her around me? Frank gently closed her eyes, and the three of us wept over her as she left us for her new life. The wonderful charge nurse, who had been sitting on a chair at the end of Tarry's bed the whole time, comforted us and then sent us home while Tarry was attended to.

The family all returned together at 3:00 pm that afternoon, to see their Tarry, who was laid out in her splendid new party dress, a white rose from one of my friends in her hands, and the little gold and diamond ring swimming on her finger. And this was exactly how she would be when she was cremated. Her brother and sisters were distraught to see their beloved sister so still, so pale and so cold. All of us had been prepared for her death, but it was a terrible shock.

My dearest wish had been granted. Tarry had died in peace and love and joy and free of all pain. I felt at peace myself. A very real sense of peace seemed to pervade my whole being. I thanked God for all this, and Cardinal Newman too.

All Caroline's wishes would be carried out to the letter; and there were no regrets. Her Requiem Mass was a wonderful and profoundly moving tribute to a truly beautiful young person. The morning of the Mass we all stamped our hands before leaving for the church. It created a very special bond between all of us who had been left behind by the "President" of that special club marked by the sign of "Tarry's tats."

Three priests, dear friends of ours, concelebrated this Mass of thanksgiving for her short, but bountiful life. It was superbly and tenderly done. The children had composed the Prayers of the Faithful. They were very up-front about AIDS in their wording. They prayed and thanked the staff at Fairfield Hospital on behalf of all AIDS carers, and of all AIDS patients. They ended with a hopeful prayer that one day a cure would be found for this truly terrible disease.

Frank had prepared the most touching, thoughtful and thought-provoking speech of farewell to his beloved Caroline. He turned to face the huge congregation and delivered this spectacular eulogy at the end of the Mass. It was so moving, and quite unexpected. When he had finished, loud applause broke out all around the church. Everyone was clapping. I have heard applause at weddings before, but never at a funeral. It was amazing.

At the end of the Mass, before Frank delivered his last farewell to Tarry, Jamie read clearly and firmly the following reflection. It was written in 1910 by Henry Scott Holland, who was the Canon of St Pauls Cathedral in London. So poignant and beautiful was it that I have included it in full.

Death is nothing at all. I have only slipped away into the next room. I am I and you are you. Whatever we were to each other, that we still are. Call me by my old familiar name, speak to me in the easy way which you always used. Put no difference in your tone, wear no forced air of solemnity or sorrow. Laugh as we always laughed at the little jokes we enjoyed together. Play, smile, think of me, pray for me. Let my name be ever the household word that it always was, let it be spoken without effect, without the trace of a shadow on it. Life means all that it ever meant. It is the same as it ever was, there is unbroken continuity. Why should I be out of mind because I am out of sight? I am waiting for you, for an interval, somewhere very near, just around the corner. All is well.

I draw comfort from this every time I read it, which is quite often.

Caroline was then driven off in her rose-covered coffin for cremation, and for the subsequent ceremonies for which she had asked. Her wake afterwards was of course at home, and our many friends were very kind.

On the next day Margie, Dominique and I took some of the large number of floral tributes over to CCU, for the staff and patients at Fairfield Hospital who had been her friends. It was eerie and strangely silent. We collected the rest of Caroline's belongings, and as I passed her room, I noticed that it had become sterile and neat again. I peeped in. The autumn leaves had gone. The bed was turned down in anticipation of the admission of a new patient that day. There was no end to this litany of AIDS.

Chapter 13

จ

Rock Pools, Blue Skies, and Golden Daffodils

It has taken a long time, much courage and many tears on everyone's part to accept this change in our lives. We were always a close family and now we are even closer.

Gradually, peace and harmony have returned to our homes. Caroline's bedroom is now the nursery for our three lovely, cherished grandchildren, Greta, Jack and the recently arrived Thomas James Hurley Mitchell. They love to stay with their Nanna (me) and Grandpa (Frank). They laugh and play with Caroline's old toys from her childhood days. These toys are placed in baskets, sit on shelves or dangle from the large windowsill. Caroline's treasures from all her travels are carefully displayed on higher shelves. She will always be with us.

When we are at Portsea, I sometimes sit on the marble edge of Caroline's grave, watching my husband tend the pots of roses planted there. I lean my back against the headstone, all warmed by the western sun, and I can hear the ocean crashing around London Bridge, not far away perhaps sweeping her ashes in and out with the changing tide.

I am so fortunate to have been Caroline's mother. She was a unique and wonderful young woman. I loved her so much and I admired the courage and dignity she displayed during her long battle with AIDS, a disease that chose a young, lovely and unsuspecting girl to destroy with stealth and viciousness. I am absolutely convinced that Caroline was spared much more suffering as a result of the love, care and comfort of her friends and family. Love truly conquers all.

The threads of my life are being re-woven to strengthen me so that I can turn to the needs of the rest of the family, who have been kind enough to tell me that they never felt neglected. They were all so patient with me during the really trying times of Caroline's illness.

Best of all, the rift between Frank and me has been mended. We are friends again. It is a great feeling to love again. AIDS, and our inability to help each other deal with it, was the thing that had come between us. It was our lasting love for Caroline and each other that healed us again when AIDS was no longer a part of our lives.

As I write these last few lines of this epic journey through and beyond AIDS, I am looking out the dining room window at the golden poplar tree. Under that tree, the daffodil quilt is coming into bloom again. I must go outside and have a look. Thank you God, and thank you Caroline.

> A quilt of daffodils grows soft and gold
> Embroidered on green grass above the cold.
> A quilt of God and nature's own design
> Was planted by my daughter, Caroline.

Epilogue

⟡

Frank's Farewell

On behalf of Joan and the family I express to you all our sincere thanks for your attendance today. We also extend our thanks to our host, our parish priest, Fr Duggan and Fr Philip Kennedy and Fr Peter Wood, who have concelebrated. We particularly appreciated the thoughts expressed in Peter Wood's homily. I would like to especially thank the many friends who have supported us in so many practical ways over the last few days.

As I sat down last evening a little after 9:00 pm to think about what I should say today, I felt quite strongly the presence of Caroline at my shoulder. I can even now hear her voice,

"Hey Dad!"

"Yes, what is it Tarry?"

"Dad, just keep it simple."

"Yes darling, of course," I replied.

My wish today is that I shall do just that. Even were I capable of it, rhetoric and eloquence have no place here. It would be quite out of keeping with the essential purity and dignified simplicity of Caroline's personality to mar her farewell to us, and ours to her, with any taint of pedantry or sophistry.

"Yes, I hear you Tarry. 'Cut the crap,' you say. OK."

Now let me first explain a few things about the arrangements today.

Following the final prayers and commendation, Caroline's body will be taken to Springvale crematorium by our friends from Tobin Brothers without escort. Caroline wanted to be cremated and we are all happy that her disease-ravaged body will serve as a source of incense rising to Heaven just as the ashes do from the thurible.

She always loved a party and you are all invited to her last party at home following the departure of the hearse. The caterers are waiting.

Let me further tell you of the arrangements.

There is a custom in the Church (of which Tarry whispers to me that she has never heard) which is referred to as the "Month's Mind." A part of the grief that the family feel at the moment is the absence today in Spain of our dear friend, Fr Gonzalo Munoz. Joan was speaking to him yesterday and he is due to be back at St Francis Church about the 19th of June. About a month from today he has agreed to bless Tarry's ashes and, with the family and perhaps a friend or two, inter them in the family plot at Sorrento cemetery. In accord with her wishes, some of the ashes will be cast into the ocean at London Bridge, Portsea.

Some of you would have recognized in the music today a few bars from a popular tune of the late Sixties. Caroline, who discussed her death and funeral several times with her mother, wanted that tune played today. I can still hear the five of them singing wildly verse after verse in the back of the station wagon on the way back from the beach at Point King, where as children they spent so many happy, sunny care-free days with the Silks, the Pleasances, the Kevins, the MacNamaras, the McCanns, the Furnells, the Clemengers, the Douez, the Donovans, the Dixons and a host of others. It is now six weeks ago that Tarry and I spent three days and two nights together at Portsea. She was very weak and I often had to carry her to the car, but I shall always cherish that time we had with each other. I would drive her to the back beach where she loved the sights and sounds of the ocean, where London Bridge was her favorite spot.

That then will be the "Month's Mind."

So much for the arrangements.

Let me now proceed to my second theme and I preface this with due notice that at times I am speaking for Caroline, at times for Joan and myself, at times for the family, at times for you and at times for myself alone.

My second theme is a litany of heart-felt gratitude — *cor ad cor loquitur* — let heart speak to heart. No, Tarry, that is not crap. Let John Henry Newman and Beethoven have some small part in the proceedings.

The first name in this litany of thanks is Joan's. I want to thank her for the beautiful gift which she gave to me on January 23, 1961; Tarry's birthday, the second of four other such gifts. I want to thank Joan too for being the wonderful mother she has been to Caroline – and I can hear Caroline's echoing cheers - and particularly for the love, comfort and solace which she has extended to Caroline in the last weeks of her short life, and most particularly in the last hours. Caroline says "thank you Mum for helping me to die so happily and so peacefully." Next in this litany are Kristen, Jamie, Margie and Dominique, and of course Sally and Peter, not to mention without dire consequences little Greta and Jack Francis. Tarry says "thank you for all your love" and the echo rings back "I love you all."

Next I turn to her legion of friends, and they were a legion. They extended from Tibet to Guernica, from Algeria to Nicaragua. Tarry left her footprints in all the continents. But I particularize here only one group whose steadfast friendship extended from kindergarten days to today. They are called simply the "card girls." Their names appear in the press obituary columns and we thank them from our hearts.

Next in this litany of thanks are her carers, and Tarry and I do not differentiate between the bodily and the spiritual carers. The contribution of each merged in a magical way. We think particularly of the staff at Fairfield Hospital in Wards Four and Five and especially in the Continuing Care Unit. No names, but to each and all, including fellow patients, our profound thanks. On the spiritual side Tarry especially wanted me to thank Fr Peter Wood, who gave her the Sacrament of the Sick a week or two ago.

This litany is not finished but I will leave the most important to the epilogue.

My third and final theme, Caroline herself, and this I must remind you is not a eulogy but the simple truth.

Like all human beings Caroline was a trinity. For centuries people have struggled mentally with the concept, the mystery of the Blessed Trinity. To me this is a complete exemplar of the tyranny of words. When we speak of three persons in one God, what does the word "person" mean, whether in English, Greek, Latin, Aramaic or Hebrew. The being that we knew as Caroline Hurley was body, mind and spirit. I want to speak of the spirit mainly. Hers was once a beautiful body. It was horribly ravaged by this disease. Her mind was rapt in artistry and the imaginative, and largely survived the onset of the virus. Joan and I can claim some responsibility and renown for the body and mind, but the spirit of Caroline was God's creation.

Let me return to simplicity.

Tarry's spirit was characterized by a sensitivity to all things beautiful. She loved all of nature, the warmth of the sun, the glories of the heavens, the sounds of the seas, the peaks of the Andes and the Himalayas, the depths of the valleys, the currents of the streams and most of all the people and the creatures of the earth. She had one (and only one) addiction – that of adventure. She lived life to the full and was little short of brimful of courage, hope, charity, dignity and generosity. She was not religious in the formal sense, but her spirit was most certainly of God's creation.

Now let me proceed to my epilogue.

A little over two years ago, with Joan, I made a pilgrimage to Birmingham, England to the Edgbaston Oratory, and in Cardinal Newman's private chapel I asked on Tarry's behalf for his intercession with the Eternal Father for a special grace – and I have prayed that prayer morning and night since. The prayer was not for a special event but simply for a special gift of grace for Caroline. The grace that I sought for Tarry was not actual or supernatural, but simply what for me grace means – the fuel that powers the spirit. I recognize that like all grace, that fuel is a completely unmerited gift from God.

I close my litany by giving my final thanks to Him, in whose house we now are, for answering my prayer.